CW00474100

Raising Your Coeliac Child

What you need to know

Lucy Nixon

Raising Your Coeliac Child

Contents

Introduction

This book is written for people caring for children with coeliac disease. It's based on our twenty years of experience in bringing up a coeliac child.

Our daughter was diagnosed aged 1, and she's now a happy and healthy 21-year-old who can cook, who knows how to manage her diet, and isn't afraid to eat out or to travel, whether she's doing a four-day hike here in the UK or spending several weeks in foreign countries.

We're based in the UK, so some of the detail may be different in your country, but the issues are the same. How do you deal with the diet—and what about all those other little (or not so little!) issues that come up every day?

If you're wondering how to start, and how you're going to manage, this book is for you. It isn't a recipe book, or a book about nutrition; it's about raising your coeliac child, and I hope it will make your life (and theirs) a little bit easier.

I'm going to refer to this condition as coeliac disease. In America, it is called celiac disease; it's the same thing. You'll see both spellings across the internet, so don't worry about it: they mean the same.

And please note that I am not a doctor, and am not offering medical advice. This book simply describes what we've learnt, in the hope that it helps you.

How to use this book

People picking up this book will be at different stages in their understanding of coeliac disease and of the gluten free diet.

So I've split the book into sections. You don't have to read from front to back!

1. The effect of the diagnosis

About the impact of a diagnosis on you, your child and the wider family.

2. Staying safe and healthy

Dealing with cross-contamination, hazards, myths and misunderstandings.

3. Dealing with the detail

Managing school, social events, travel and making mistakes.

4. Coeliac disease and the gluten free diet

Symptoms, what is (and isn't) safe to eat, reading labels, weaning and prescriptions.

5. Practical matters

Useful lists and documents.

From the beginning...

Imagine: it's 3 in the morning, it's dark outside, and it's very, very quiet. We're on holiday in a tiny studio flat in an isolated block of flats by the beach on an unmade road. Our 1-year-old daughter is awake and screaming inconsolably.

We're used to her being up early, and being awake in the night, and to taking it in turns to try and calm her and get her back to sleep.

But we're in a foreign country, and feel bad about our neighbours. So we try everything we can to settle her (clean nappy, milk, rocking, stories, songs), including making up a bowl of Weetabix, in case she's hungry. Little do we know that this is the worst thing we could be doing for her...

Nothing works, in any case, so we put on our shoes, and take her away from the flats, walking away down the unmade road, in the dark with our screaming child.

Unexpected problems

She was ill for months before we realised there was a problem. It sneaked up on us.

Once she was weaned, she vomited at almost every meal. But babies do vomit a lot, don't they?

Her dirty nappies were awful: the wrong colour, wrong smell, wrong consistency—and far too many of them. But she was our first child, and we didn't know what to expect.

She sat on the floor and played quietly where she was, while the other children crawled over and under things, exploring their surroundings. But some children are late to crawl; and she was very good at jigsaws.

She didn't sleep well, waking early in the morning, and during the night, often crying, and always with a dirty nappy. But she'd been a colicky baby, and we were used to broken nights, especially since we also had a newborn.

She slipped down the growth charts at the baby-weighing clinics. Her feet didn't grow for months. But it happened slowly, slowly—and neither of her parents are particularly tall.

I visited my parents, who lived several hours drive away, and my mother (who trained as a nurse) was a very hands-on granny. When she changed my daughter's nappy, she immediately said "this isn't normal". This started the series of doctor visits.

Luckily for us, our family doctor at the time was very experienced and decided to test for three different things, in order: giardia, cystic fibrosis, and finally coeliac disease. Stool tests, sweat tests, and blood tests... and then a biopsy.

While we were waiting for the tests, and then for the results, (which took nine months) the relentless vomiting and diarrhoea continued.

It got worse.

She started developing a pot belly. By now her arms, legs and buttocks were very skinny, and we had to go down in nappy sizes, until at 20 months she was wearing the same size nappy as her 3 month old sister. Those tiny nappies didn't do a good job at all, and I did a lot of washing—of babies, of bedding, of floors, and of clothes, hers and mine.

She gradually started refusing most food.

This, of course, was coeliac disease. Unknowingly, by giving her Weetabix, bread, and other food typically eaten by infants and toddlers, we were increasing her pain, and making her illness worse.

What was that again?

You may have been so bemused by the announcement that you didn't quite catch the words the doctor used. Or perhaps you need to explain it to someone else... again. You're going to do a lot of explaining over the next few years!

The condition is called coeliac disease and it is pronounced SEE-lee-ak (emphasis on the first syllable). Sometimes it is known as gluten-sensitive enteropathy, or coeliac sprue, but it is all the same thing, and not fun at all.

What is coeliac disease?

- It's an autoimmune disease caused by the immune system reacting to gluten
- It's surprisingly common: it is estimated that about 1 in 100 people have it, though not all of those are diagnosed
- It is a lifelong condition—your child won't grow out of it

- There are a lot of different symptoms, and some people have 'silent' coeliac disease, and don't show any symptoms
- The only treatment available at the moment is a gluten-free diet for life
- It is hereditary, meaning that it runs in families. People with a first-degree relative with coeliac disease (a parent, a child or a sibling) have an increased chance of developing it themselves.

What is gluten?

Gluten is made up of two proteins found in wheat, barley and rye: gliadin and glutenin. These grains are ground to make flour, and that flour is used to make a wide range of different products such as bread, cake and pasta.

Wheat, barley and rye are very commonly found in our western diets.

- Wheat is often found in bread, cakes, sauces, cereals and pasta
- Barley is used in malt, soups, malt vinegar, cereals and beer
- Rye is also commonly found in rye bread, cereals and beer.

And gluten, of course, is therefore very common indeed.

When it is mixed with water, gluten forms sticky strands. These strands bind things together, and trap air bubbles. Kneading traditional bread dough (or rolling and folding the dough many times, if you're making a puff pastry) helps create these sticky strands, and helps trap air into the mixture. The results are therefore light and airy and can be formed into wonderful shapes. Think of a croissant!

This explains why gluten free breads can be hard and heavy, and can crumble badly—though this is getting a lot better these days. It just means that different techniques and ingredients need to be used to make gluten free bread.

Because of its special properties, extra gluten is sometimes added to bread dough (in addition to the gluten already there), or to other food products, to help bind them together or to help them keep their shape.

What is the problem?

When someone with coeliac disease eats gluten by eating wheat, barley or rye, it triggers an immune response that damages the lining of the small intestine.

The lining is covered with villi: thousands of small finger-like bumps or stalks that enormously increase the surface area of the inside of the small intestine (think of carpet pile). And the villi are covered in microvilli (like shaggy hairs on each of the villi), which further increase the surface area.

Nutrients are absorbed via the villi. Eating gluten causes an immune reaction which shortens, or even flattens, the villi. This reduces the surface area of the small intestine, which means that nutrients can't be absorbed properly. This in turn means that the person may suffer from malnourishment, and is at risk of suffering from conditions caused by malnutrition.

Sometimes people debate the term; is it desirable to call it a disease when it isn't contagious, and (when it is properly controlled by diet) you feel perfectly healthy? An alternative is to say coeliac condition, but that can sometimes sound a bit vague. Another issue is the 'suffering' word. Do you say 'I suffer from coeliac disease'? Again, this may not be true, if you are maintaining a strict diet, as you may not be suffering at all. Apart from doughnut deprivation, of course.

We tend to go for 'she is a coeliac' if the situation comes up—along the lines of 'he's a diabetic'.

What is dermatitis herpetiformis then?

15-25 percent of people with coeliac disease typically have no digestive symptoms, but do have an extremely itchy skin rash. This usually appears symmetrically (left and right sides) and often appears on the elbows, knees, buttocks, back, face or scalp.

We don't have any experience of dermatitis herpetiformis, but I understand that it is unbearably itchy and has been described as "...like rolling in stinging nettles naked with a severe sunburn, then wrapping yourself in a wool blanket filled with ants and fleas...".

Dermatitis herpetiformis is diagnosed with a skin biopsy (they only take a tiny amount of skin, and it doesn't usually leave a scar).

Treatment for dermatitis herpetiformis is a strict gluten free diet, and usually (to start with) treatment to help reduce the severe itch.

12

A small percentage of people with coeliac disease suffer from dermatitis herpetiformis as well as the typical digestive problems seen in coeliacs.

What causes coeliac disease?

Coeliac disease often runs in families, and research shows that it is linked to the HLA-DQ2/HLA-DQ8 genes. However, many people have those genes without having coeliac disease. So there must be more to it, but what?

There are a variety of theories about what triggers the development of coeliac disease:

- Some experts think that stressful events such as surgery, severe illness, emotional stress, menopause or pregnancy can trigger the disease
- It has been suggested that extended use of some medicines, such as antibiotics, can act as a trigger
- Some research suggests that gastrointestinal viruses (e.g. rotavirus) can trigger it too
- Some scientists think that the increased rate of coeliac disease could be due to the increased gluten content in our diets over recent decades.

And some think it is none of the above.

What is clear is that gluten in the diet is a key element of developing coeliac disease. If you've never eaten gluten, you wouldn't develop coeliac disease.

Researchers across the world are working on coeliac disease, looking at:

- Preventative measures such as vaccinations to avoid people developing the condition

- Treatments such as pills, or ways to adjust someone's microbiome (the bacteria that live in the intestines) to help people stay healthy if they have developed it.

However, the only treatment available at the moment is a strict gluten free diet—for life.

The effect of diagnosis

Not yet diagnosed?

If you think your child may have coeliac disease, then do consult a doctor to get them properly tested. It may not be coeliac disease, and if you treat them for coeliac disease and it isn't, they may not get proper treatment for the real problem.

If your child is still going through the diagnosis process, then please don't remove gluten from their diet yet. If you do, then their gut may start to heal, and the true situation may not be revealed to their doctors. I know it's hard to see your child suffering but this matters.

As soon as you have the diagnosis, you can eliminate all gluten from their diet. We were advised to wait to see a dietician before removing all gluten, which we did. I think we should have switched our daughter to a gluten free diet immediately, and if I had to do it again, I would. The change in her was astonishing, and we could have saved her a few weeks of pain.

Newly diagnosed?

You finally have a diagnosis; something that explains why your child has been unwell. Or maybe it's come out of the blue, and your child has been diagnosed with coeliac disease while being investigated for something else, and they aren't showing any of the classic coeliac symptoms.

You probably have mixed feelings; possibly a mix of:

- Relief (at last you know what the problem is—particularly if you've struggled to get a diagnosis)
- Guilt (where did they get this from? It's genetic; is it my fault? Why didn't we notice earlier?)
- And panic (what am I going to feed them?).

You may be in denial.

Just as there are said to be five stages of grief when someone you love dies—denial, anger, bargaining, sadness and acceptance—there are different stages of grief when you (or someone you love) receives a diagnosis of chronic illness. And you may experience each of them at different times.

Denial

"This can't be happening to us... she's fine, surely? Nobody in my family has this problem; there must have been a mistake."

This is a particularly likely reaction if your child has silent coeliac disease, and isn't showing any symptoms.

Anger

"Why does this have to happen to us? Why is it so difficult?"

It is hard, at least to start with, while you are getting to grips with the new way of life. And your child (if they are old enough to remember another way of life) may be angry that they can't have the same food as their friends. But you can do it—and it could be a lot worse! I used to tell myself that 'it is only coeliac disease' and remind

16

myself that there are many, many worse problems she could have.

Bargaining

"Maybe when she gets better, she'll be able to eat some normal food" or *"maybe just a bit of birthday cake at parties"*.

Thoughts like these are natural; moving your child to a gluten free diet is a big step, requiring significant changes to the household. You'll need to tell yourself (and others) that this wish for what has gone must not be acted on. Eating gluten when you have coeliac disease damages your health with every bite.

Try learning as much as you can about coeliac disease. The more you know, the more in control you'll feel.

Depression

It's normal to feel sad about the diagnosis, and about the necessary limitations to your child's life. Not only will your child not be able to eat quite the same foods as everyone else, but their children too may have the same problems.

Sharing food can be a vital part of social interaction; it is fundamental to life, and your whole approach to feeding your family will have to change.

Try one or more of the following:

- Join your local support group, so that you and your child can learn that you are not the only ones dealing with the issues

- Look for foods that they can eat, and which they like—experiment with the new food alongside them, recognising that they won't like everything
- Learn how to prepare and cook a range of gluten free meals; once you have some control back, you'll feel better able to deal with the diagnosis
- Don't give up!

Acceptance - it is true and I can cope

With luck, when the symptoms have subsided and your child begins to show some enthusiasm for life again, you'll be able to accept this new way of life.

This is the goal. It doesn't mean that every day will be easy, or that you'll never be sad or angry about it again; it means that you've understood that you can do it, and it will be fine.

Remember: a consistently gluten free diet for the whole of life is currently the only treatment for coeliac disease. But if your child can stick with the diet, their chances of remaining healthy are as high as anyone else's.

You can do this.

What now?

I was overwhelmingly relieved when we finally got a diagnosis of coeliac disease. Our daughter had been tested for cystic fibrosis, which would have been much harder to deal with. So I was relieved that it was 'only' coeliac disease, and very pleased that we knew what we had to do to make her feel better.

But it isn't easy at first, and so I strongly recommend that you look for support. This could come from a variety of sources:

- The national group for coeliac disease in your own country. Here in the UK, it is Coeliac UK, but many countries have one or more such national group. Coeliac UK is a campaigning charity, dealing with legal and medical issues, increasing awareness and supporting its members, and funding research. I highly recommend joining such a group, as they have a lot of information that will help. Here in the UK, for instance, Coeliac UK produces a book every year (and updates to this book every month) containing lists of foods that are safe to eat. This is extremely useful, and we took it everywhere with us

- The local group. Here in the UK, Coeliac UK has local groups in many areas. These groups meet regularly for fun, to share information and maybe food, and to learn more about living with coeliac disease. These local groups can be a great source of local information—such as which restaurants are good for coeliacs—and often have a lot of expertise in dealing with the diet. And sometimes it is good to talk to people who understand the problems you are facing, because they've dealt with those kinds of problems themselves

- Online. There are now many online groups, such as forums and Facebook groups, where you can learn more and get help. Just bear in mind that occasionally people in such groups have other motives for being there. There are groups for everything: I recently joined a Facebook group about gluten free fish and chips, and another one about gluten free beer. The information is out there!

- Friends and family. Do talk to your friends and family about what it is like, and how you feel about it. They'll need to know anyway, to know how to help and what to feed your child

- And if there isn't a local support group, or if the one that exists doesn't suit children, why not volunteer to run events for locally diagnosed children? When our daughter was diagnosed, it was relatively rare for children that young to be diagnosed, and the local group was quite grey-haired. I found it very helpful indeed to talk to other parents of children diagnosed young. And (as she got older) our coeliac was glad to know that she was not the only one. Many young children and teens need not to feel different, or singled out; they want to know that they fit in.

Don't forget: a diagnosis like this affects the whole family, and not just in practical ways such as finding a dedicated cupboard for gluten free food, or changing the way that you eat. It can have a psychological impact too, bringing up some strong emotions. It could affect siblings (who may feel jealous that their sibling is being treated as 'special') as well as adults, who may feel angry, guilty or depressed. Any or all of the family may struggle with the diagnosis, either immediately or over time; it doesn't just affect the one diagnosed.

Something to bear in mind

Families which are proactively engaged in managing the disease tend to have children who become more adjusted to the diet (more likely to stick with it, and not cheat) than those who don't.

And those children are likely to stay healthier.

That's worth aiming for, so come up with some plans to help the family adjust. For example:

- Thinking about meal plans
- Rearranging the cupboards
- Researching coeliac disease on the internet
- Going to a support group event (such as a gluten free Christmas party for children).

The beginning of recovery

How quickly will we see a change?

There's no guarantee; it will depend on each child, and on how ill they were—and what their particular set of symptoms were.

We saw a difference after a couple of weeks of putting our daughter on to a gluten free diet, when we saw an extraordinary improvement in her health and energy levels—and she asked for food.

This tiny girl who had refused food, gradually reducing her diet to small portions of spicy sausages, grapes and milk (all gluten free, now I think about it), who regularly vomited up what little food she did eat, and who was unable to get the nourishment she needed from our everyday meals—now wanted second helpings.

It makes me want to cry even now, 20 years on, just thinking about the first day she asked for food.

It took a while for her body to adjust. From being a typically malnourished one-year-old (stick arms and legs, no bottom and a distended stomach), she went to being a chubby—even chunky—two-year-old. At this point, a doctor who hadn't seen her before expressed surprise that she was a coeliac; of course, as we know, coeliacs can present with a variety of different issues. He was clearly expecting the malnourished version.

We believe that this phase was her body's reaction to the near-starvation of malnourishment; piling on the pounds in case the famine happened again.

That changed over time. Now she is a slender young woman (and has been for many years). She is shorter than average, which may be related to the malnourishment as an infant; but her parents aren't tall, so who knows?

You may be wondering whether the risks of further health issues associated with coeliac disease are reduced if your child successfully sticks to a gluten free diet. The answer is that they are.

Try not to be overprotective

It may be difficult for you to believe that everything is going OK.

You've probably taken your child to lots of appointments, and watched them go through lots of tests. Maybe you've had to help hold them down so the doctors could take blood, or put a tube down their throat. Perhaps you've watched as your child's health gradually deteriorated. Maybe your child was one of those with behavioural problems due to eating gluten.

You'll probably see improvement in their health—and maybe even in their behaviour too—as a result of the change.

And because your whole family is learning how to navigate this new gluten free lifestyle, you're likely to be watching your child for health issues, and monitoring their diet very closely. You'll no doubt assume that any little blips (minor illnesses, tantrums or irritability) are due to gluten having crept in somehow. Or that any health issues your other children have are also gluten-related (they could be; but they might easily not be anything to do with gluten).

All this is normal. And it is important that your child understands that the gluten free diet matters. But they do need to learn how to handle it themselves when they are old enough, because you won't be there to manage their diet all the time.

It needs to become normal in their mind, and in yours. Not 'the same as everyone else'—because they aren't the same—but completely normal, and not something to worry about.

After all, they are different. But no more different than people who can't eat peanuts, or who don't eat meat at all, or who keep kosher, or... Differences in diet are normal.

And the number of people diagnosed with coeliac disease grows all the time, meaning that almost everyone knows of someone who doesn't eat gluten. It gets easier all the time to find gluten free food; it really will be OK, as long as they can keep to a strict gluten free diet.

Benefits of sticking to a strict gluten free diet

We know that it isn't always easy in the early years, but once you've got used to it, it really isn't that hard. And the benefits are immense.

Not only should your child become happy and healthy again, with energy to learn and play as they should do, but you are also ensuring that they don't develop other long-term, life-changing, and even life-threatening conditions by continuing to eat gluten.

Untreated coeliac disease can lead to a range of problems, such as:

- Rickets in children (bone softening and weakening)
- Osteoporosis in adults (loss of bone density)
- Nervous system disorders
- Pancreatic problems
- Cancers of the mouth, oesophagus, intestines, liver and lymph glands
- Anaemia
- Chronic diarrhoea
- Chronic fatigue
- Infertility (in men and women)
- In women: delayed menstruation, premature menopause, miscarriages
- Emotional problems, such as irritability and inability to concentrate
- Weight loss.

Please don't worry; I've included these just to make it clear that the gluten free diet really does matter for coeliacs.

So do keep your coeliac child on a strict gluten free diet, no matter how hard it seems, or how great the temptation to let them cheat. Once they've been on the gluten free diet for a while, their risk of suffering from these problems is no greater than anyone else's risk.

Think positive

It is sometimes very hard to be different. And it can be difficult to watch your child deal with feeling different and with (sometimes) feeling excluded. It is hard to watch your child missing out on some treat that others are sharing.

But there are some good things about having been diagnosed with coeliac disease.

1. There is a diagnosis. You know what the problem is, and you know how to help your child feel better. There will be difficult days, but you know what to do.

2. Your child is lucky to have a diagnosis; many people suffer for years before they are diagnosed, which can lead to all sorts of other issues.

3. Your child will feel better—healthier, and with more energy—quickly, and will be 'normal'. It is wonderful to see your child start to join in with games and activities that they didn't feel up to before. Our coeliac daughter couldn't join in with the activities at Tumble Tots because of her lack of energy before diagnosis, but she soon started to cause the havoc that small children do, with her younger sister as accomplice. She is now fit and healthy, and swims regularly at university.

4. Your child may well end up eating a healthier diet than before, if you (and they) can cook from scratch. Avoid using too many processed gluten free foods as they can often be high in fat and sugar to compensate for the lack of gluten.

5. It's 'just' a change in food. Yes, I do know it isn't easy, but there are no pills or injections needed to make them feel better.

6. You become part of a community. It may not be one you wanted to join, but it is amazing how many times I've had a conversation with other shoppers in the free from aisle of a supermarket. That kind of community just doesn't happen by the tinned tomatoes!

Practical tips

Be prepared

Always plan ahead.

Depending on the age of your child, and therefore how long they can wait to eat, be prepared to carry gluten free snacks around with you. You may not always be able to buy something suitable in a hurry.

Be prepared to discuss your child's dietary needs with many people, whether you are booking a holiday, thinking about school, going out to eat, sending them to Scout camp... you will develop a set of phrases that work for you. I tended to say something like:

"My daughter has coeliac disease. This means she will be ill if she eats wheat, oats, barley or rye. Can we talk about how to manage her diet while she's with you?"

I've included a draft letter at the end of this book which you can copy (and change) to send to whoever you need to explain the gluten free diet to.

Living gluten free is getting easier every year, and more people know about coeliac disease. But there are still people who don't really understand what it means, or how important it is to avoid contamination, or who haven't heard about it before at all. You will be explaining it to a lot of people—and that's a good thing. Every time you explain it to someone new makes life easier for all the other coeliacs out there.

How to survive the first year of living gluten free

Has your child just been diagnosed? Here are some tips to help them—and you—get through that first year of being gluten free.

1. Be brave and optimistic. It will be difficult, but your child will feel better as their intestine heals. And your child will take their lead on how to feel about their diagnosis from you—if you despair, so will they.

2. Clear out some cupboard space, dedicated for gluten free products. They can be very bulky, especially if, like me, you feel you have to buy everything you see to encourage the supermarkets and manufacturers to keep making/stocking it. If you have gluten products in the house that nobody else in the house eats— bin them. Don't let your child eat them just to avoid waste.

3. On the other hand, it's important to recognise that just because something is gluten free, it may not be good to eat, and your child doesn't have to like it. We have tried some awful gluten free products in the past...

4. Join the local support organisation, even if you're not a natural joiner. Here in the UK, it is Coeliac UK. They will have advice, tips and other helpful material. Coeliac UK produces a list of manufactured foods that are acceptable for coeliacs to eat, and offer updates every month. If

there are local meetings—go to them! And talk to people, no matter how shy you feel.

5. Read every label. On everything. Labelling has got a lot better, but sometimes manufacturers change the recipes of your trusted favourites, so don't assume it will be gluten free forever. If you're not sure, don't let your child eat it—and contact the manufacturer to ask if it is OK. Working out what can and can't be eaten will become easier as you learn what can instantly be discarded, leaving you to concentrate on the things that might be safe to eat.

6. If you're in the UK, carry the Coeliac UK book of food and drink that your child can eat around with you. You'll be surprised how often you use it.

7. Learn as much as you can—even if you end up knowing more than the local doctor does. Your doctor, after all, has to know something about a lot of things. You can concentrate on what affects your child. Then you'll be able to assess whether they will be able to eat codex wheat, lactose, oats...

8. Find other people in the same situation. We went to local meetings but when there wasn't a local support group for children, we set one up. It helped us a lot in the early years to talk to other parents in the same situation. If there isn't a local group, then these days there is the internet.

9. Don't ever be persuaded by people saying "just one [cream cake, doughnut, slice of quiche] won't

hurt". It will, even if your child can't feel any difference. It will be eating away at their small intestine, and set their recovery back. Don't do it.

10. Do be prepared to explain it often, and sometimes over and over again. No it is not a fad; yes it is a medical requirement. The number of times you have to do this may mean your child comes to dislike eating out because of the embarrassment factor, especially as they enter their teens—eating in places that have dedicated gluten free menus will help.

11. Be prepared to be pushy—you will have to ask what is in dishes, and double-check if necessary. But do be polite. You don't want them just to pick the croutons out of your child's portion of soup or salad, and give them the same bowl again, leaving the crumbs in!

12. Do avoid cross-contamination. Some people set up dedicated areas in their kitchen for gluten free food preparation, with dedicated chopping boards, knives, pans etc. Even if you don't go this far, do think about a dedicated toaster (or buy lots of foil for the grillpan), a dedicated gluten free bread bin and even separate pots of butter, jam etc. Don't forget to label them clearly, and tell people why. It only takes someone to dip a knife with gluten crumbs into the butter for your child—and, inevitably, you—to spend the night in the bathroom.

13. Do plan ahead for festivities and celebrations. From Valentine's Day to Mothering Sunday, Thanksgiving to Christmas, school trips to birthday parties, celebrations involve food and drink. Plan ahead—what will you and your child eat?

14. Consider travelling and days out—an emergency travel pack of gluten free snacks can be invaluable!

15. Don't forget drinks—these can contain gluten too, whether they are alcoholic or soft drinks. Be careful.

16. Don't get complacent—check every time, as recipes and cooking arrangements can change.

17. And at the end of the year, celebrate! (With something gluten free, obviously).

Family matters

It is important that your child understands that she has coeliac disease (even if they aren't old enough to call it that yet) and that there are some foods that other people can eat but which will make them poorly.

If your child is very young at diagnosis, then they probably won't be able to remember being able to eat whatever they wanted—but then, they won't remember being ill, either.

Children who are old enough to remember eating, say, an authentic croissant, or chocolate brownie icecream, may struggle to give these foods up—but they may remember how ill they felt before diagnosis too, which could be an incentive to help them stay on the diet.

But not everybody experiences symptoms that made them feel unwell before diagnosis—even though gluten would have been causing internal damage. These children may need some extra encouragement to stick to the gluten free diet.

What to say to your child

I was horrified to read about a family where the child was not told of her diagnosis immediately; nor did they switch her diet immediately. Every gluten-containing meal she ate was damaging her unnecessarily.

So do explain it to your child in a way that they'll understand.

Our coeliac daughter was diagnosed aged 1; we used to talk about her 'special tummy' when talking to her, and to talk about coeliac disease when explaining it to others. She picked up the proper words when she was old enough.

It is important not to make a fuss about the diet, but to treat it as a normal part of life. Treat it seriously, because strict compliance to the diet matters to their future health, but it's not a drama. Your child will need to learn to cope on their own as they get older, and you really don't want to introduce issues around food.

If you need help with explaining what coeliac disease is to your child, there are child-friendly books available for children of different ages.

We talked about how everyone is different—some have red hair, or need glasses, or have legs that don't work so well—and having a special tummy is just one of the things that is different. But the best thing is, in our view, simply to keep the messages simple, talk about it when relevant and don't talk about it when your child doesn't want to. There will come a time when it is simply too embarrassing to be discussed *every time* you eat in public. (With luck, the teenage embarrassment won't last too long!)

Don't make food a stressful situation for your coeliac child, or at least minimise the stress. Dietary issues are stressful enough on their own. If your child is also aware of your stress and worry—for example at eating away from home, perhaps at a friend's birthday party—it will raise their levels of stress, reduce their pleasure in eating and in the experience as a whole, and may cause some food-aversion in the future. Bear in mind that what you find OK to talk about may still be acutely embarrassing for your child.

Don't make them feel that the gluten free diet is difficult, or that it makes life more difficult for you. Obviously it does make things more complicated, and it can be more expensive—but don't let them know that, because that's too much of a burden for a child. Knowing that the diet has its downsides may make them think that they shouldn't stick to the diet, in an attempt to be helpful to you, and that would obviously have an impact on their health.

Keep it calm.

Explaining to others

Keep it simple. Not everyone needs to know everything there is to know about coeliac disease. All you need for them to know is how to help keep your child safe and healthy.

Tell them that your child has coeliac disease and must keep to a strict gluten free diet to stay healthy.

You can tell them that it is an autoimmune condition.

Do tell them that it is not the same as a peanut allergy; eating gluten won't mean a trip to A&E except in severe cases of allergy, such as anaphylactic reaction to wheat. But do make sure they understand that there will be consequences. We found that explaining that it will trigger vomiting and diarrhoea is usually enough of a warning for them to be careful! No parent wants your child to vomit at their child's birthday party…

And do tell them what your child CAN eat. Keep it positive.

These days almost everybody will know of somebody with a food allergy or intolerance, and most will be sympathetic.

Talking to guests

It may seem awkward, but it is also important to explain to guests in your house the meaning of the labels on the various pots of food, and the purpose of different utensils (for example, if you have a dedicated bread board for gluten free bread, you don't want a helpful guest setting out gluten-full bread on that board).

We recently failed to explain things to a new guest, and had to re-allocate a block of cheese that had been intended to be gluten free, but which had been put down on a board with gluten-full bread crumbs. It wasn't his fault; we hadn't told him. But that cheese couldn't be used for general cooking, either, because cooking doesn't remove the gluten from food.

How family members may react

Your family members will probably react in a very similar way to you, experiencing emotions from disbelief to acceptance. They may also, surprisingly, feel some jealousy that your child is 'special' in some way.

Their feelings may be complicated by the fact that there is likely to be a genetic aspect to coeliac disease, and this could well affect them too.

Getting others tested

If any one of your immediate family—not just a child, but also a parent or a sibling—has been diagnosed with coeliac disease, it is important that the rest of you get tested, as there is a significant chance that other people may have it as well, as it is an inherited autoimmune disease.

There have been lots of studies that show that the likelihood of a first-degree relative having coeliac disease is higher than in the general population:

- An identical twin has about 70% chance of also having coeliac disease
- A brother or sister with the same tissue type has about 30-40% chance
- A brother or sister who doesn't have the same tissue type—about 10%
- A child—about 10%
- A parent—5-7%.

Are my other children going to have the same problem?

Not necessarily, but they might. If you are worried, have them checked (and yourself). And don't forget, even if you've all been checked once, and the results were negative, any of you might develop the problem later.

How it affects siblings

I invited our non-coeliac daughter (we have three children, only one of whom is a diagnosed coeliac—

though our second daughter has been tested for coeliac disease a few times) to tell you how it was—and is—to be the sister of a coeliac.

Being the sister of a coeliac was definitely difficult for me at times, especially as a child. Not nearly as difficult as it was for her of course, but it had small effects on me and my brother. Why does she get special food? How come her food gets a separate cupboard? Why aren't I allowed to eat that? But it became normal as I grew up with it. We're best friends of course, but sometimes I was jealous of her. I wished I had coeliac disease. She got all this different food, she got to go out to 'gluten free food tasting things' with my mother, she got more attention because she was 'special'.

I often got told off for asking her why she couldn't take one bite—not even a crumb?—because I didn't understand the effect it would have on her or how little it takes to make a coeliac ill. Now I'm a teenager, I know why she gets different food, and often more of it, but it was hard to grasp this concept as a young child who couldn't quite understand invisible illnesses.

Each time someone at school said the word 'gluten' or 'coeliac', I'd jump at the chance to tell everyone about my sister and her 'special tummy'. She'd feel embarrassed sometimes when she had to bring her own food to a party, and everyone 'watched' her. It was even worse when people offered her food and, feeling rude, she had to decline, simply because she couldn't eat it. These people would almost always have a moment of realisation a few seconds later and fuss around her, offering her this and that and she'd try to hide from all the attention.

I can see why she gets so excited when she discovers a new occurrence in the gluten free world—Warburtons making gluten free bread, or new discoveries such as gingerbread men, or even, more recently, puff pastry. And I can understand her disappointment when supermarkets make the gluten free section smaller at Christmas to make room for all the gluten filled produce on their shelves.

I realise I take these things for granted and often forget that she might feel resentful that she doesn't get to eat the same food as us. Not that she would, she's hasn't got a jealous bone in her body. Perhaps it's the gluten free diet that makes her more understanding. She'd always listen politely while I complained about my brother scoffing our entire packet of biscuits and how she was so lucky to not have to share. She'd just try to convince me to go gluten free.

How it affects adults in the family

It isn't always easy for the adults in a family either. Things that we've found difficult include the following.

Making a fuss

Trying to keep our coeliac daughter safe when eating out, while not 'making a fuss' or embarrassing her in public. Sometimes your child just won't want to hear you explaining the consequences of eating gluten, yet again, to a stranger.

Keeping things 'fair'

Trying to make everything 'fair', when it isn't possible. For example, not buying treats because they're not gluten free can lead to resentment from non-coeliac siblings; or buying them for the non-coeliac children, but not being able to find a gluten free equivalent, meaning that the coeliac is left out, again.

This one is a balancing act, and the trick is to know what the coeliac's favourite things are. Maybe there aren't any gluten free doughnuts, but she does really like Jelly Tots.

Dealing with disappointments and near misses

A couple of times, after careful checking and consultation with the staff, our daughter has been presented with food only to have it whisked away before she started eating it (or, worse after she'd started to eat it) because the staff have suddenly discovered that it is not gluten free after all. Better that they do take it away, obviously, but the adults then have to deal with the disappointment of the child, and their own frustration.

Dealing with the fallout

Sometimes things go wrong after a series of bad choices.

Once a teacher suggested that our daughter's physical reaction to having been given (and having eaten) the wrong food on a school outing was psychosomatic.

A few times our daughter has fainted on school trips because she hasn't eaten (because she wasn't given food she could eat, and she didn't like to ask or make a fuss).

This is frustrating for parents; but making a big deal out of it won't help anyone, and a child has to learn to manage away from their parents. There are two things here: educating the adults caring for your child, and ensuring that the child has some backup food supplies for emergencies.

Getting it wrong

Guilt when you get it wrong: when she was a lot younger, our daughter was given the wrong pizza once (we failed to label it correctly). She ate it. Afterwards she said that she'd thought it looked unusual, but that she'd thought 'why would they give me pizza that wasn't OK for my tummy?' The guilt still stings...

Assuming you're getting it right

Once you relax into the diet, it's all too easy to lower your defences and forget to check something yet again. That's when mistakes are made. Yes, we've done that one too. More guilt.

The trick here is to remember that both parents will make mistakes. Just because your partner got it wrong today doesn't save you from making another mistake tomorrow, so don't beat them up about it. Try to make sure that everyone learns from each mistake, so that at least it will be a new mistake next time...

Practical tips for family

If people in your extended family are reluctant to accept the dietary needs of your child, you could try the following:

- Cook for them (rather than have them—fail to—cook for your child). Yes, this means you'll have to take on more tasks, but it might help in the long run. They might see that gluten free meals can be delicious
- Be the one who offers to make the (gluten free) Christmas cake, or to bring something gluten free to the party. Be prepared to remind people every time until they've got it; and offering to bring gluten free food can be a polite way of reminding people
- Offer to cook together; that way you can see what is going into the meal, and where the cross-contamination risks might be, and you can explain why you do things a certain way (foil on the grill pan, and so on)
- Asking about ingredients in a meal (or asking to read the packet) can also serve as a reminder. If you can do this in advance, they may remember not to add the croutons to the salad, or to offer ice cream wafers on the side, rather than stick them decoratively into the ice cream... Sometimes it's just those little changes that make all the difference.
- And they won't know, for instance, that their brand of stock cube may have gluten in, or that soy sauce (usually) contains gluten. Those things that become second nature to you will be news to others.

- Show them articles in the media about coeliac disease occasionally. It's odd how the written word can seem more official and believable than the spoken one
- Consider writing them a letter to explain about coeliac disease and the need for a gluten free diet. Perhaps they didn't really understand and don't like to ask. Having something written down means that they can take time to reread it
- If you have to, and can do it without worrying your child, you could explain about the consequences of eating gluten for your child in the longer run. Granny might care rather a lot that your coeliac daughter may have trouble conceiving a baby if she continues to eat gluten!
- Do remember to emphasise that this is a medical condition, diagnosed by specialists, and not any form of faddy eating.

Be prepared to explain, and to keep on explaining. Most people don't know anything about gluten or coeliac disease, and it can take a while for people to accept that there's a problem. It will take even longer for them to remember not to double-dip their knife in the butter (leaving crumbs). You will eventually learn a simple script to help explain the situation in a clear and objective fashion.

The gluten free diet is also, of course, probably not playing as big a part in their lives as it is in yours. Where you will learn to read every label, and to question every dish, before offering it to your child, they've got their own problems to deal with, and just may not be focused on yours.

It may be that it brings up issues in their own lives. Because food plays such a large part in our social lives, it gets very tangled up with emotion, and it can sometimes be difficult for people to be entirely rational on every occasion. And sometimes people are afraid of illness, or afraid of change, or afraid that your child's diagnosis may mean that they should look at their own food choices too.

You may find individuals who refuse to eat gluten free food. We went to a child's birthday party where the hostess had carefully provided gluten free food so that our daughter could eat without worrying... one woman chose to refuse the party tea, and to take her children to McDonalds instead, saying "my children don't do gluten free". It was very rude, but it was her problem, not ours; nobody has to have gluten in their diet.

Staying safe and healthy

You know that coeliac disease is a lifelong condition, for which the only treatment at the moment is a strict gluten free diet. If you can help your child stay on a strictly gluten free diet, then their health should be good (in this respect, anyway!)

But it isn't always easy. There are several potential pitfalls:

- Denial
- Cross-contamination
- Hidden hazards
- Misunderstandings and myths.

Let's look at these in turn.

Denial

I mentioned denial as one of the stages of grief, earlier.

It is a major threat to keeping your child healthy and safe on a strict gluten free diet.

Denial of the diagnosis

You (or your child, or your family) may deny the diagnosis.

"It's not true; it's a mistake; she doesn't have the classic symptoms; it doesn't run in my family (or his); the results were inconclusive; she'll grow out of it."

No, she won't grow out of it, and if you have a diagnosis, you have it, no matter if you don't have the classic symptoms.

You (or your child, or your family) may be ambivalent about the diagnosis, choosing to succumb to temptation, and the kind of thinking that could make your child ill:

"Just one biscuit won't hurt"—yes it will. Every bite is causing internal damage, even if you aren't aware of it.

"But it's my birthday"—even more reason to treat yourself well, surely?

"Don't be mean, let her share the cookies"—this diet is not a fad but a medical necessity. Would you knowingly offer a child food containing poison?

"It says low-gluten"—yes, but low isn't the same as no, is it?

Denial of the need to be tested

Your family may be in denial about the need to be tested. It's a genetic condition, after all, but some people refuse to be tested. Or they were tested once, and it was negative.

Adults have the right to make their own decisions about their health. You can't make someone get tested, though you can explain the situation to them. It's their health; their decision.

Denial that this is a serious condition

Some people deny their symptoms are severe, choosing to ignore the problems.

Some people say that they couldn't manage the diet.

Or they say *"just don't tell the doctor"*; but it's not the doctor's body; it's your responsibility to teach your child how to stay safe.

Another comment could be: *"I know other coeliacs who eat this"*. My response would be to say "more fool them, then", but a more helpful response would be to say "that's their choice and their body that will be damaged".

This kind of denial isn't helpful. Obviously you can't make someone get tested, but if your relative is negative about the diagnosis, the symptoms, or the difficulty of managing the diet in your child's hearing, then your child may well pick up on this and decide that if it's too hard for Auntie Mabel (who is a grownup) then it's far too hard for them (because they're just a child). You may need to ask Mabel not to comment.

It's just a fad

People around you may deride the gluten free diet as a fad. This is an odd form of denial; it is true that there is a trend for people to eat gluten free by choice, but for those with a diagnosis of coeliac disease it is not a fad but a medical necessity.

I've got mixed views about this. It's great that the gluten free market is booming. It means that there are a lot more options for coeliacs than there used to be. On the other hand, if someone is half-hearted about being gluten free then it makes it less likely that someone who genuinely needs to be gluten free will be taken seriously.

Cross-contamination

We all do it, even if the best etiquette manuals say not to: using your own knife or spoon to dip out some butter or marmalade. If that knife has just spread butter on your 'normal' bread, and then you dip it into the marmalade—or back in the butter—the chances are high that you've just added some crumbs with gluten into the butter or marmalade. If the next person to take some butter happens to be gluten free, you've probably just given them stomach pain, diarrhoea, wind (and maybe worse).

What if you cut 'normal' bread, and then cut cheese with the same knife? What if you stir a pan of 'normal' pasta, and then stir a pan of gluten free pasta with the same spoon?

Other potential sources of cross-contamination include toasters, grill pans, bread boards, colanders, sieves, baking trays, leaking bags of flour on supermarket shelves—or in your own cupboards—scoops used in pick-and-mix sweetie counters, or in health-food stores, putting croutons on a salad and then just taking them off to make it 'gluten-free' (or buns on burgers, wafers in ice creams...), or even just passing some 'normal' bread across a bowl of gluten free soup and getting crumbs in the soup.

If someone in your house has to live gluten free, the best way to avoid this kind of problem is to make sure that they have their own pots of butter, jam, mayonnaise or whatever, clearly labelled. You then have to be sure that all visitors to the house understand the rules, too! It took our daughter a long time to discover that she liked jam—and that was once we bought a set of tiny pots of jam for her to taste. She used to eat her bread dry... was it because she was worried about cross-contamination?

Lucky coeliacs have enough space in their kitchen to have a dedicated gluten free area, with their own implements, or families that all go gluten free together. Everybody else—with less space or money—has to be very vigilant, to be sure that if a spoon or knife has gone into something that contains gluten, that it goes nowhere near the gluten free foods. If you're cooking both gluten-containing and gluten-free things in the same oven, use different baking trays. Don't put pizza directly on the oven shelves unless you're going to wash them afterwards (which shelf had the normal pizza on? Will you remember which it was in a week?). You can use foil to make a protective barrier between the oven shelves and the food, or on baking sheets, or to create individual 'trays' for cooking on. And put the gluten free food above the gluten-containing food in the oven, cupboards and fridge.

Using a fan or convection oven? These work by blowing the hot air around the oven; great for even heating, but that does mean that they're also blowing tiny particles of food around—and that could include gluten-containing flour particles. My oven does both fan and standard cooking, and I never use the fan option.

Keep things clean: microwaves, ovens, work surfaces, tools, cutlery drawers...and your hands.

Buy a second toaster. Have you seen the crumbs that accumulate inside a toaster? Or you can toast under the grill (remember to use that foil, though) or, you can buy Toastabags—these are great, and will protect your slice of toast from other crumbs.

What about when you go out to eat? There is a reason why McDonalds say that coeliacs shouldn't eat their fries if they have a special promotion on for some other gluten-containing treat—oil is easily contaminated. Tiny pieces of crumb coating or spices can float free of one item and land on another.

Just as risky is the idea that simply taking the bun off a burger, or the croutons off a salad will remove the risk of gluten contamination. Obviously that's better than eating the bun/croutons, but there will be some crumbs left.

Lots of factory-produced items now say 'Produced on a line [or in a factory] which also processes nuts, gluten, celery... [add in your own allergen here].' There is a risk—probably tiny—that gluten could be transferred from one item to another in the factory, and the manufacturers are covering themselves.

Only you can make the decision about whether to take this last risk—and making decisions about your child's health is so much more difficult than with your own. Only you can assess how sensitive your child is to gluten, and it does seem to vary from person to person. We tend to accept this risk, and our daughter eats items with this warning without a problem; but your experience may be different.

But it does make sense to avoid cross-contamination as much as possible at home.

Should everyone in the house go gluten free?

It's an option, of course, and one taken by many; but it is an expensive one. We run a mixed house, because there are five of us, and we manage it very carefully.

I do cook more dishes than I used to that are completely gluten free (or can be made gluten free) so that we can all eat the same, such as fish pie, or risotto. I think sharing food is important; and I don't want our coeliac daughter to feel more different than she needs to. But I do sometimes find that I'm making three trays of lasagne, for instance: a normal one, a gluten free one, and a vegetarian one.

And sometimes a recipe is better for being gluten free. Our gluten free brownie, for instance, is better (in my view) than when I make it using 'normal' flour. And some top chefs are recommending gluten free flour over 'normal' flour for making batter.

You may find, though, that it is easier in your circumstances to go completely gluten free in your house. That's fine, of course, and makes it easier to for your child to stay gluten free at home. However, you may have to make a special effort to teach your child how to manage to stick to the diet when outside the home—and you may experience some resistance from any other non-coeliac members of the family.

Hazards

Gluten hides in all sorts of places. I can't possibly list them all here, but here are some hazards that we didn't expect to come across:

- Soy sauce (choose tamari, but still check carefully)
- Spices (sometimes have flour in to prevent caking, or as a bulking agent)
- Baking powder (sometimes has flour in as a bulking agent—look for ones using gluten free flours such as rice flour)
- Stock cubes (some brands are not gluten free)
- Dried yeast (some brands of dried yeast contain wheat starch)
- Smarties (the coating shell has gluten in it)
- Some yoghurts and ice cream (obviously ice cream with cookie dough or chocolate brownie in will contain flour, but so do others, and some low fat yoghurts use gluten—presumably as a binding agent to hold them together)
- Some cheap, low-fat cream cheeses are thickened with wheat starch
- Chips (french fries, if you're American) and other processed potato shapes or even pre-prepared roast potatoes can be dusted in flour to make them crispy when cooked
- Some wafer thin meats have a dusting of flour on to help the meat slices separate nicely

- Some bags of pre-grated cheese are dusted with flour to help the cheese gratings stay separate (grate your own: it's cheaper anyway)
- Marzipan (in some countries, such as America, it may not be gluten free)
- Some cloudy fizzy drinks (gluten may have been added to make it cloudy)
- Some fizzy drinks (barley malt colouring / flavouring)
- Some herbal tea bags are sealed with glue containing gluten
- Drinks from drinks machines may contain gluten—particularly if you're requesting hot chocolate—and there is a general risk of cross-contamination from the nozzles.

We have always been careful about:

- Glue (for example, on envelopes and stamps, though we've never come across a problem)
- Play-dough (you can make your own, which works well, but doesn't last as long as shop-bought).

Are there risks in going gluten free?

There is certainly a risk that your child ends up consuming more calories: often gluten free processed foods have extra sugar and fat to compensate for the lack of gluten and to add taste.

There may be a risk that cutting out food without considering good replacements means that some nutrients may be missing from your diet, though this is true of all food groups. For example, most standard breads and cereals are made from flour that has been fortified with folic acid, iron and B vitamins; naturally gluten free flours are not usually fortified. The best way to ensure that your child gets all the nutrients they need is to encourage them to eat a wide variety of foods: fruit, vegetables, nuts and seeds, meat and fish, eggs and dairy.

But you can safely remove gluten from your child's diet (or your own!). You do not need gluten for a healthy life.

What about shampoo or bath products?

Sometimes people worry that they shouldn't use products such as shampoo or conditioner if they contain wheat (or barley, etc).

This is a personal decision, and everyone's experience is different. But gluten-containing skin care products and cosmetics aren't a problem for coeliacs unless they are swallowed. Gluten can't be absorbed through the skin.

So just consider whether there is a risk that your child is going to swallow some of the product. Toothpastes (at least here in the UK) don't contain gluten—but lipstick might.

And if your child does have a skin reaction to a skin care product, don't forget that this could be due to an entirely different allergic reaction, not necessarily due to coeliac disease.

Myths and misunderstandings

There are many myths surrounding the gluten free diet. The biggest ones we've come across are:

1. They'll grow out of it

No. If you have coeliac disease, it is a lifelong condition. It is true that for some people there may appear to be a remission during the teenage years, and for some people it can take a while for symptoms to reappear, but it is dangerous to assume that you can therefore eat gluten. Gluten causes internal damage.

2. A little bit won't hurt

Yes it will. You may not see an immediate effect (though many do!) but there will be damage to the lining of the small intestine.

3. You can burn off, or kill, gluten with heat

Heat does not get rid of gluten. Oil that's been heated hot enough to fry gluten-containing food in will still contain tiny gluten-containing crumbs for the next fry-up. Use fresh oil. Nor does gluten burn off in a pizza oven or on a griddle.

4. You can't have coeliac disease if you are overweight

Yes you can. An undiagnosed coeliac could be fat or thin; suffer from diarrhoea or constipation (or, indeed, have symptoms that are completely unrelated to the gut).

5. A gluten free diet helps you lose weight

Only eating less and exercising more helps you lose weight. Often foods that are specifically prepared to be gluten free are high in fat and sugar; and some foods that are naturally gluten free aren't necessarily good for you either.

6. Coeliac disease isn't life-threatening

It isn't life-threatening in the way that a peanut allergy is life-threatening. However, the consequences of untreated coeliac disease can be life-threatening, long-term.

7. Coeliac disease is rare

Not really: it is estimated that 1 in 100 people have coeliac disease. That's over 10 people in an average secondary school.

8. Coeliac disease is an allergy

It isn't. It is an autoimmune condition, in which the villi in the small intestine are damaged.
There is such a thing as gluten intolerance (not the same as coeliac disease).

And there is a gluten allergy (again, not the same as coeliac disease). In this case, someone will experience an allergic reaction (e.g. swollen lips or difficulty breathing).

9. Only old people have coeliac disease

Not true. Our coeliac daughter was diagnosed aged 1, and she isn't unusual. You can develop coeliac disease at any age.

10. Gluten free food is healthier

It can be; often coeliacs cook from scratch, so they know what is in their food. This kind of cooking often can be healthier.

But manufactured gluten free food often isn't better for you than 'normal' food, as it can contain lots of fat and sugar to make it taste better. For example, comparing a well-known brand of gluten free white sliced bread with a well-known brand of white sliced bread reveals that the gluten free bread contains 6.1g of fat per 100g, while the normal bread contains 1.7g of fat per 100g. Read the label.

11. You can diagnose gluten sensitivities yourself

No. Go and see a doctor.

You could cut gluten out of your child's diet without seeing a doctor, of course; but without a diagnosis you won't get prescriptions for gluten free food (which would be free for children here in the UK); any future tests for coeliac disease would be inaccurate because of the gluten free diet; and gluten may not be the problem in the first place—your child could have other problems.

12. Coeliac disease is curable

No it isn't. It is a lifelong condition, and at the moment the only treatment is a strict gluten free diet. People are investigating vaccines and other treatments, but there isn't anything available yet.

Tips to avoid contamination

We don't run a completely gluten free kitchen. This means that we have had to think carefully about contamination.
We use:

- a gluten free cupboard for bread, flours etc
- a gluten free bread bin
- a gluten free biscuit tin
- lots of foil
- dedicated pots of butter and jam (labelled)
- and dedicated knives/serving spoons/boards at table.

We don't have a separate toaster any more, because we learned that our coeliac daughter doesn't much like toast. If she wants toast, then we put foil on the grill pan, and make toast under the grill. It's probably best to have a separate toaster if you think you'll toast bread a lot.

We are always careful not to pass 'normal' bread) over the top of other food or drink (or pl etc).

We label things carefully—usually just with a marker pen, but sometimes with sticky labels. You can buy special ready-written labels, but you don't need them. Mistakes happened in our house when we didn't label as well as we should have.

And don't forget to explain to people that they can't put a knife that's just spread butter onto a 'normal' slice of bread into a pot of jam that is dedicated to the gluten free eater.

On storing food: lessons we've learnt

If you don't label something that you put into the freezer 'for later', then you'll probably have to throw it away 3 months later because you can't remember what it is, and whether it is gluten free or not. So you end up discarding it to be safe...

Cake storage tins and biscuit tins (and toasters!) collect crumbs, often in fiddly places it is difficult to keep clean. I do recommend dedicated tins to keep things separate.

I'm even careful about which bag I pack what into at the supermarket. 'Normal' bread from a bakery (even in a supermarket) usually comes in a loose bag with tiny airholes, or in a brown paper bag. These will leak crumbs onto other foods.

Do try to find space, even if it's only a shelf or a drawer, to dedicate to gluten free food. Make sure that it is higher than the gluten-full food storage space. Not to make it more difficult for your coeliac to find their treats, but because bags of flour inevitably leak and you don't want gluten-full food to fall on top of gluten free food or on to plates and bowls stored underneath.

Your coeliac will appreciate having their own cupboard full of things they can eat (rather than having to look through all the things they can't). Put the biscuit tin for any non-coeliacs on the other side of the kitchen, and make sure the tins look different (even if you've labelled the tins, pre-reading children may get confused).

Your dedicated cupboard for gluten free supplies will probably always be too full. You'll collect free samples to try, and will experiment with different gluten free ingredients, and will probably buy new gluten free products to try just because they're new. Try to find a big cupboard if you can!

Have periodic clear-outs. We get samples from allergy fairs, and when we see new products we buy them for our daughter to try. She doesn't like everything. So we end up with plenty of out of date items that won't get eaten. If you can find a coeliac friend who'd like to try them, so much the better!

On breadmakers

You can buy a wide variety of different gluten free breads these days, but if you choose to make your own, do invest in a breadmaker with a gluten free programme. Baking gluten free bread isn't the same as making your own 'normal' bread, and while you can make your own by hand very successfully, if you're going to bake bread often, then a breadmaker might just make your life easier.

Practical tips when cooking

- Do the gluten free version first. If, for instance, you're making two lasagne dishes (one gluten free, one not) then layer up the gluten free lasagne version first, so that you're not touching one, then touching the other
- If you're baking, use paper cake tin liners to line the (clean!) tins, because crumbs can lurk in crevices
- If you're making two kinds of pasta (normal and gluten free) then ALWAYS drain the gluten free pasta first—it makes sure there are no mistakes, and saves on washing up. Better: consider separate colanders and sieves (because you know how difficult it can be to clean those thoroughly!)
- If you're a big toastie-making family (or waffles or...), then you'll probably need two toastie-makers (waffle-makers, etc) to be sure that one is completely gluten free
- We use a lot of foil to cover baking trays / grill pans etc—and it reduces washing up!
- Wooden spoons can harbour all sorts of things if they have cracks in. Keep an eye on them, and replace with plastic if necessary.

Medical issues

Although there is initially a vast improvement in the quality of life in the first year after diagnosis—as reported by patients—after that, there is a steady decline in reported quality of life in adults and adolescents aged 8-16 diagnosed with coeliac disease, quite possibly due to poor self-management.

The issue appears to be that in some cases (apparently especially for women) suffering a chronic condition increases anxiety and depression.

Once diagnosed and on a gluten free diet, the level of anxiety decreases.

However, if people find it difficult to maintain the diet, especially outside the home, then this can lead to increased anxiety, leading to the coeliac trap:

feeling unwell – diagnosis – gluten free diet – anxiety – poor self-management – feeling unwell ...

Not surprisingly, parents of coeliacs also report increased anxiety, and a study found that children report more problems of distress and impact on their lives than parents are aware of. (Learning that could be the cause of even more parental anxiety, of course).

A key factor in achieving a good quality of life is believing in one's own ability to manage the diet. If someone understands the issues and know how to manage the diet, they are likely to have a better quality of life.

Counselling might help those people who struggle at managing the diet, in an attempt to break the cycle. If this is you or your child, then don't be shy of reporting this to your medical professionals; they may be able to help, and this might make things better in the long term.

Ongoing testing

Once your child has a diagnosis of coeliac disease, you'd hope that there'd be some kind of ongoing testing, to make sure that all was going well. This may well vary by country, and, here in the UK, it seems to vary by area too.

Our daughter was under the care of a general UK paediatrician, and had blood tests every year until she was too old to see the paediatrician, and was discharged back into the care of her GP. The blood tests were a general check on health, but also to check that she was following a truly gluten free diet.

At the annual paediatric checkup (until she was 16), she was weighed and measured, and asked questions about her diet, her bowel function and (as she got older) her experience of puberty. Very embarrassing for a young teenager!

She also had annual bone scans for the first 10 years, to check that her rate of growth and bone density was satisfactory.

This may not be the experience of every child; among other things, it will depend on the availability of dedicated paediatric gastroenterology clinics near you. We didn't have one.

She also received some gluten free food on prescription from her GP. This is a difficult issue in the UK NHS at the moment; prescribing practices are very different in different areas. If you are in the UK, then do check the Coeliac UK site for your area, to find out what the provision might be.

Other testing

You may be interested in supporting research studies. We've done several. For example, donating blood to a study of the relationship between thyroid problems and coeliac disease, and—more recently—supporting a psychology student in studying the issues around young people with coeliac disease transitioning from paediatric services to adult services. If you're interested in joining research studies, contact your country's coeliac support organisation (in our case, Coeliac UK).

Growing up

Not surprisingly, the psychological study we were involved in found some issues around the transition from child services to adult services, mostly to do with a lack of information and an abrupt reduction in support.

If your child is coming up to 16 years old—especially if they were diagnosed recently and so are still getting used to their new lifestyle—and is discharged from paediatric care to their GP, they may feel unsupported. This could lead to struggles with managing, and sticking to, the gluten free diet. Here in the UK, you as a parent may find that your child is expected to take on full responsibility for managing medical appointments, prescriptions etc, and that you are no longer in control of these things—and yet your child may still need support.

Be aware that a poor experience of this transition between services can lead to your child/young adult disengaging from the support available to them. Make sure that your child/young adult knows that even if they've not been transferred to an adult gastroenterology service they can get help from their GP who can refer them to an NHS dietician or to gastroenterology services if need be. And, of course, there is support available from Coeliac UK and from similar organisations in other countries.

Medical care

It is likely that you'll be concerned over every illness and ailment that your child experiences over the next few years, from dentistry to diarrhoea. Of course, some of the issues might be due to gluten; but many will be completely independent.

You will probably find that you mention coeliac disease to a whole range of different medical professionals, just in case it's relevant.

For example, our daughter broke her scaphoid (it's a small bone in the hand) by falling off a bicycle while we were on holiday. After a visit to A&E, it turned out that there was an area of weakness in the bone... was this due to coeliac disease? Probably not, but it could have been. It is important that coeliacs are aware of the risks of osteoporosis, and keep to a good healthy diet.

You should know that virtually all medicines prescribed in the UK are gluten free. A few contain wheat starch; if a medicine contains wheat starch, it will say so on the label. You'll have to get into the habit of always reading the label, just in case. If you are concerned, your pharmacist will be able to advise you.

Prescriptions

Here in the UK we are very lucky that some basic gluten free staples are currently available on prescription—items such as flour, bread, pasta, pizza bases, crackers and a few plain biscuits. However, it is getting more difficult as certain areas find that they have to cut back on issuing prescriptions for gluten free food. Indeed, there is (at the time of writing) a consultation over whether gluten free products should be available on prescription at all.

It does cost money to get prescriptions filled—in England, but not in Wales—but in certain circumstances the charges are waived, including:

- if you are under 16, or under 19 and in full-time education
- if you are 60 or over
- if you (or your partner) gets certain benefits
- if you have an NHS tax credit exemption certificate
- if you have a prescription exemption certificate.
- You can get a prescription exemption certificate (ask your doctor or pharmacist) if:
- you are pregnant or have had a child in the past year
- you have one of a range of medical conditions, such as diabetes or epilepsy.

- You may also be able to get the prescription charge reduced:
- by buying a 'season ticket' (Prescription Prepayment Certificate—ask your doctor or pharmacist)
- or if you have a low income. This will depend on your circumstances—ask at the social security office or hospital or call the NHS.

If you have to pay for prescriptions, it is definitely worth buying a season ticket, as this will significantly reduce the cost to you over the year. And of course, it will be valid for any prescription during the time it is valid, not just gluten free food.

Dealing with the detail

Classroom life

Dealing with school meals

School meals are a problem.

In theory, at the time of writing, here in England (and in some other countries) all state-funded schools are obliged to make arrangements for supporting children with medical conditions—and free school lunches should be offered to all pupils from Reception to Year 3 (inclusive).

And yet, the provision of a gluten free school meal still seems to be a problem.

My daughter ate a baked potato for lunch every day for the final 7 years of her schooling. And we sent her in with a packed lunch for the first 7 years, because at her school, they would only arrange for a meal to be sent in from some central department, with no guarantee that it would be at all similar to what the others were eating that day. We decided that since she was different enough already, this would only emphasise the difference. So many people eat packed lunches, that this would be a good way of ensuring that she wouldn't look too different.

This will vary enormously by school. Some schools seem only to offer dinners, and don't allow packed lunches; others are the other way around. Some school catering teams are very enthusiastic about the challenge of providing gluten-free meals; others don't want the responsibility. Some invite you to send in food for them to reheat.

We recommend talking to the Head and to the catering staff—and maybe to the school governors as well. You may need to make a fuss; it won't be for the first time (or the last) I'm sure.

Treats from teachers

Some teachers like to offer sweets, either as regular treats for good behaviour or work, or as gifts at Christmas or for birthdays. Always talk to the teacher at the beginning of the year, and if this happens in their classroom, send in a pack of gluten-free sweets for them to have to offer your child.

Baking and other activities

This will depend on the age of your child. Be aware that play-dough is not gluten-free, and nor are some glues. You can make gluten-free play-dough if necessary.

Children may do baking at nursery or school—this is clearly a contamination risk. You could send in special flour (don't forget to send gluten-free baking powder as well), and you will need to check the other ingredients; for example, writing icing for decorating biscuits may not be free from gluten.

I suspect that children at nursery do still make pasta pictures, too. You could offer a pack of gluten free pasta to the teacher, just in case your child decides to try eating uncooked pasta covered in glue and paint...

Birthday cakes and other special events

Sometimes children bring in cake or sweets as part of a celebration—perhaps of their birthday. There is always the risk that these may not be suitable for your child. Some schools don't allow this kind of sharing, or find a way of reminding carers and students of the various allergies that have to be managed at school.

If you can, talk to the teacher about how the school likes to manage this, and if need be, you could provide the teacher with a pack of suitable gluten free treats that could be offered to your child instead.

Do be careful about taking in gluten free cakes or biscuits to be shared with the class. Sometimes gluten free sweet treats just don't taste the same as 'normal' ones, and it would be counterproductive to have the rest of the class reject the gluten free versions brought in by your child. If you're confident that the class won't be able to tell the difference (and there are some amazingly good cakes and biscuits available to be bought now, and some excellent recipes) then that's fine, of course.

And on the subject of being prepared...

When discussing your child's condition with your teacher, consider letting the teacher know that sometimes the child might need to go to the toilet urgently. Reminding your teacher of the unpleasant consequences should certainly be an incentive to ensure that they are given permission to go when needed.

On the tiny number of occasions when our coeliac daughter had a gluten mishap, she was too ill to go to school anyway. But if the consequences of a gluten mistake should hit while your child is at school, you'll want them to be able to go to the school toilets as needed.

School trips and other residentials

Day trips

You will need to discuss this with the teachers. I always sent packed lunches for these trips, but I have been caught out when one of the activities was 'cooking in the Victorian kitchen'—which involved kneading bread. Make sure that hands get thoroughly washed!

Residential trips

If you are sending your coeliac child off on a school residential course or other camp, you may be worried about keeping them gluten free. Here are some things to think about...

How sensitive is your child to cross-contamination?

Some people seem to be more sensitive to this than others, and it is something to bear in mind when planning the trip. Obviously you will be alerting the carers to cross-contamination issues, but they do need to understand the importance of this.

How far away are they going? Could you easily rescue him or her if they fell ill?

Clearly any child could fall ill on a trip, but it has to be said that those with chronic conditions that are vulnerable to the environment are more likely to have a problem—including asthmatics and diabetics. It is no fun to be ill away from home, particularly if there is the ongoing risk of further problems because the caterers haven't properly understood the issues.

How long are they going for?

You might be able to send foodstuff for two or three days, but if it is longer then you will almost certainly be relying on others to prepare and cook meals for your child.

Is it literally camping, or is it somewhere with trained caterers?

In theory, trained caterers should be aware of the issues, but this isn't always the case. Check!

If it is camping, there will be constraints over availability of preparation space, cooking utensils etc, and possibly an increased risk of contamination as a result.

Is it a destination where just your child's group will be present, or will there be other groups there too?

Going to a location where just your child's group will be there offers a better chance for control of the environment than if they are going to a large mixed venue. On the other hand, if it is a big place, used to catering for lots of people, they are more likely to have come across the need for a gluten-free diet before.

How much responsibility does your child take for their own diet?

It can be difficult for a child to say to a relatively strange adult "I can't eat that" or "please don't use that spoon to serve my meal"—but this is an important skill that they will have to learn if they are to control their own diet in the future. It may be helpful to have a fact-sheet that they could hand over. This is even more important if your child is abroad and trying to communicate in another language.

Does your child know what they can or can't eat?

Again, this is something that they will have to learn for the future, and part of the point of this kind of away-trip is to increase independence in the children. This is why I think these trips are so important—and it's amazing to see how different your child seems on their return.

Is your child likely to swop food with his or her friends?

Well, do they do this at the moment? Dreadful thought...

Or are they likely to succumb to peer-pressure and have what everyone else is eating?

Children vary in how they react to peer-pressure. The problem is, if they do eat what everyone else eats and don't react, they may think it is OK to do this more often. And, of course, it reduces the importance of a strict gluten free diet in the eyes of those around them, too.

How supportive of your child's diet are the other children in the group?

If your child has been gluten free for a while, and they are going with their school, it is likely that the others in the group will have accepted that your child eats differently. But in a group of children your child doesn't know, the other children will want to know why your child isn't eating this or that. Does your child know how to explain? How will they react to any teasing?

How much trust do you place in the carers?

You will be able to assess this better if you speak to them and discuss the issues. Some people are more knowledgeable than others about gluten-free issues; some people are more open to learning than others. Ask yourself—does school/Brownies/whoever cope with the gluten free diet for your child at the moment? To avoid any doubt, you could provide a factsheet that clearly states what your child can and can't eat. (See the final section of this book for an example).

Do you even want to send food with your child?

There may be practical difficulties with sending food with your child. If your child is away for a week, any gluten free food that you send with them may have gone stale by the end of the week.

And usually, I have found, you don't get a discount for sending food with your child, so you end up paying for their food twice.

How integrated do you want your child to be with the other children?

Eating a completely different meal because you sent food, rather than a slightly modified meal prepared on site, may simply make your child seem even more 'different'.

Have you discussed the menu plan with the carers?

If not, then you should. Even if you trust them, going through every meal with them will help emphasize the importance of the detail. Remind them that snacks and sweets can be dangerous too.

Do the carers know what symptoms to look out for?

Not all coeliacs react the same way. If you make sure that the carers—and your child—know how to recognise a gluten episode in your child, then your child is likely to get care quicker. And if your child is likely to vomit at the table (as some do) it might just help focus their minds.

We sent our daughter away several times (Brownie camp, school residentials, summer camps). On each occasion, I discussed things carefully with the teachers and/or caterers at the destination. I sent her with a box of gluten free items (bread, buns, cake, breakfast cereal, biscuits, pasta, pizza base, flour) based on the menu plans, but not with pre-prepared meals. Part of the worry with pre-prepared meals is how they would travel or keep. Perhaps you could send known and trusted brands of non-perishables as an emergency supply (such as a tin of beans, snack meals).

I believe strongly that this kind of trip—without the support of family—is an important step in raising an independent adult. Your child will probably have a wonderful time, and their meals should not be the main focus of the trip—the trip should be the focus.

And if there are mistakes—unpleasant as they might be—your child will learn from that too.

School cookery lessons

Both primary and secondary schools here in the UK offer cookery lessons (and no doubt elsewhere too).

There's no reason why your child shouldn't do cookery lessons in school, as long as everyone is aware of the issues, and takes care to minimise any risk involved.

These risks are mostly of contamination due to inadequately washed equipment, shared equipment, or contact of non-gluten-free food (e.g. flour) with gluten free food, either directly or because clouds of wheat flour end up in the air due to the high level of excitement. There could also be a problem of confusion in the classroom (which tray of cakes did I make?). These could be avoided by ensuring a dedicated work area and good labelling at every stage. It may be possible to use a different shaped baking tray, for instance, or a unique shape of cookie cutter and a dedicated baking tray.

Even if your child bakes with gluten-containing ingredients in the knowledge that they won't eat the end results, there's always a risk of unwashed hands with bits of gluten-containing dough under the fingernails making their way into the mouth.

It is possible to opt to study cookery (sometimes called domestic science or food technology) and to take exams in this subject. Again, there is no reason why your child shouldn't be able to do this too. Indeed, I have been contacted a couple of times by the food technology teacher in my children's school to ask about certain aspects of cooking for the coeliac child (mine and other people's coeliac children). Often children choose to do a research project as part of these exams, and coeliac disease is a fairly common topic to explore.

None of my children opted to study food technology, but they did all have some cookery lessons in school.

Being social

Nurseries and other childcare

When she was young, our daughter went part-time to a day nursery, and we provided much of her food. I took in her bread, which could be kept frozen in their freezer, and defrosted a slice at a time for breakfasts. You could also consider providing packets of gluten-free cereal, as well. She ate the meals provided by nursery when they were OK for her to eat; I went through the menus with the cook to talk about what would and what wouldn't be OK. If the meal wasn't going to be free from gluten, I took in frozen food which could be defrosted as needed. In those days, there wasn't so much available, and I spent time making gluten-free fish fingers, chicken nuggets and 'tinned spaghetti', so that her food looked as much like the others as possible. All these things are now available at supermarkets.

As for schools, it is the unusual events that will catch you out—parties, treats and outings. You will always need to double-check that they have remembered, and will often need to send supplies for your child.

Birthday parties, school parties and discos

Children's birthday parties (and other social events for large groups of children) can be difficult.

My daughter always took her own party food with her. I discussed it with the hostess of the party, and tried to come up with something that looked as much as possible like what the other children are eating. I used to make miniature birthday cakes for her to take along as well—but I found that they weren't ever eaten, so I gave up.

These days it's a lot easier for people who are not used to the diet to find gluten free food in the supermarket, even birthday cakes these days, so you may find that they will offer to provide gluten free food for your child.

Of course, if it is your own child's party, then you can easily make the whole meal free from gluten, and their guests will never notice; though look out for small friends who might have brought extra treats along. If you are worried that a small guest may say "Yuck!" about the bread, for instance, and upset your child, you could make two types of sandwiches, and tell your child which are OK.

Party bags are a problem – you can hardly ask someone to make up a special party bag for your child. I made sure that nothing was eaten until I had checked whether it is OK or not, and had substitutes available. I found that my children always shared party bags with their siblings, saying things like "this is OK, so you can have this one ...", "this isn't, so he can have that one ...". Your child will become familiar with what sweets are OK, and which are not.

Tea and sleepovers

Your child's best friend's parents may become nearly as familiar with what is acceptable and what isn't as you do. If you are lucky, they will remember, and will provide a naturally gluten-free meal for your child. I always checked—it is difficult for a child to refuse food, particularly if pressed, as it will seem impolite. I also always offered to send supplies of special bread, pasta, flour—whatever seems appropriate.

Food swopping

We have never had a problem with this, though I can imagine that it does happen, and that some children find it difficult to resist. The gluten-free foods are often packaged in a very 'worthy' pack, appealing to an adult idea of health; a brightly coloured pack of gluten-full food, perhaps with one of your child's favourite TV characters on, may be very tempting.

All you can do is explain to your child that someone else's food may make them poorly. Good luck with this one.

Cubs, Brownies and other group activities

As for school, discuss this with the adults in charge. It is perfectly possible for your child to join in almost all activities with very minimal change. My daughter has successfully been away on Brownie and Guide camps, and much more recently she completed her Gold Duke of Edinburgh four-day hiking expedition without any issue with gluten. It can be done—with a bit of planning.

Other social events

You'll no doubt be invited as a family to other types of social events, such as weddings or anniversary parties.

Talk to the host or hostess in advance, to see whether they've made any plans for catering for your child.

If these are being held at a restaurant or hotel, or being catered by an outside caterer, you can call the catering team in advance to discuss the gluten free diet.

If the event is pot-luck style, with everyone bringing something to share, you can obviously make sure that what you bring is gluten free. And if you feel comfortable about it, call other people that you know are going, and ask what they're planning to bring. Maybe that will be gluten free too... Make sure it's something that your child really enjoys—and serve your child first, to be sure that their meal doesn't get contaminated by any mix-up over serving spoons.

Eating out

Are we ever going to be able to eat out as a family?

Yes you are! With a bit of planning, perhaps phoning ahead if you're not sure, this can be done. Your child won't have the same choice as everybody else, but they won't go hungry.

You can take your own food to some places—though beware of cross-contamination. For instance, McDonald's will put one of their gluten-free burgers into one of our bread rolls. But some pizza ovens are laden with semolina (which is derived from wheat) to stop the pizzas from sticking, so be careful where you take your pizza base. Several big-name pizza restaurants now serve gluten free pizza (such as Domino's and Pizza Express) and you can buy gluten free fish and chips. It is even possible to find some restaurants and cafes that are 100% gluten free.

The excitement of finding a place where the menu is marked up as to what is gluten-free, so that we don't have to discuss it yet again, is quite absurd—and we have decided to stop and eat at places we were passing which advertised their gluten-free food in the window or on the menu, even when we weren't ready to eat yet.

What do we need to think about?

Eating out with a child who needs a gluten free diet can be tricky. Eating out with children who don't have dietary problems can be stressful, but if you need to analyse every item on the menu as well as deal with the usual childish issues, it can be a real problem.

In fact, many adults don't eat out either, once they realise they need to eat gluten free. According to Coeliac UK, 67% of people are less likely to eat a meal outside of home once they are diagnosed.

This is a shame, for a number of reasons:

- Eating out is one of life's pleasures
- I really enjoy not just eating a meal I haven't had to prepare, but one I haven't had to think of in advance or shop for (how many meals do you know that will suit three children—not only a coeliac, but also a child who won't eat vegetables, and one who won't eat meat?)—and which I won't have to wash up afterwards
- How to behave in a restaurant is an important skill for children to learn, whether or not they need a special menu. I know it is hard work, but the more you do it, the easier it gets—honestly!
- Not eating out reinforces the view that 'there's no call for gluten free meals'. If nobody asks for them, then they won't offer them. That's the way the market works.
- Explaining to a waitress—or even to chef, if need be—about the gluten free diet makes it easier for the next one along.

I've been vegetarian for over 35 years, and the changes that have taken place over that time are entirely due to individual vegetarians asking for vegetarian food and explaining why—repeatedly. Let's do the same for gluten free!

Reading menus

Over time, you'll get the hang of quickly deciphering what menus are telling you, so you can eliminate some dishes completely, and then discuss the details of possible options with the staff.

For example, foods that are described as breaded, battered, coated or crusted are unlikely to be safe to eat unless they also say that they are gluten free.

Descriptions of meals that mention the following are also unlikely to be gluten free (unless it specifically says so):

- Pies and pasties
- Pastry
- Crumb
- Gratin
- Crumble
- Dumplings
- Yorkshire pudding
- Croutons
- Bechamel
- En croute
- Fritters
- Soy sauce
- Teriyaki sauce

- Noodles
- Pancakes
- Cake.

Things to be careful about:

- Be wary of fried foods (in case the oil contains bits of gluten-containing food from a previous meal)—and, depending on context, also check on food described as crunchy or crispy, which may mean fried. And fried and pan-fried may mean the food has been dredged in flour before being put in the pan
- Sausages and burgers should be checked, at least here in the UK, as they are highly likely to contain rusk (which is bread-based)
- Dishes that involve gravies or sauces need to be checked with the restaurant staff, as do some dressings (which could contain soy sauce) and pickles (malt vinegar)
- Also check the chips (fries, if you're American) and other potato products—check that they haven't been tossed in flour to make them crispy. We've fallen foul of this in the past, on one camping trip that was memorable for all the wrong reasons
- And check the side dishes: no croutons on salad, no wafers in ice cream. Check the sauces for ice cream too!

Think about which kind of cuisine will work well:

- Fast food: the big names (e.g. McDonalds) will give you the meat patty without the bun if you ask nicely, but beware the chips/fries in some places (e.g. Burger King), and avoid the special spicy or curly fries everywhere

- Italian: a risotto would probably be OK, as would meat/fish (check the sauces) but pasta and pizza are problematic unless they offer gluten free bases and are very conscientious about cross-contamination
- Chinese, Japanese and Thai: these can be tricky because of the soy sauce and noodles issues. But if you order carefully, and discuss with the staff, you can find food that will work. Rice noodles are fine; it's the wheat/egg noodles that you should avoid
- Mexican: be careful about the tortillas. Some are made from corn, but some from wheat. Ask!
- Indian: don't eat naan bread, samosas, paratha or other wheat-based breads. But the main meals and rice should be fine. Check with the staff
- Middle Eastern: avoid tabbouleh, because it is made from bulgar wheat. Pitta breads are made from wheat flour. Check the falafel, too. But meat and fish meals should be good (remember to check everything).

And don't assume that your child can or will only eat food from a children's menu. Often these are highly gluten-laden (pizza, sausages, pasta, fish fingers and so on), but the adult's menu will have more gluten free options. And sometimes restaurants will offer a smaller portion of an adult meal for a child; ask them. Or you could order one adult meal between two children.

Making it work for your family

If you've not been to a particular restaurant before, do consider phoning ahead to check if they can provide gluten free food—and check their website too. After a while, you'll be able to tell whether they genuinely understand about coeliac disease, or are just going through the motions.

If you can, check the menu before you arrive. Often these are available on the restaurant websites.

If you've been there before, don't assume that what your child ate last time will still be OK to eat this time. Menus change, recipes change and ingredients supplied to the restaurant change. What was gluten free last time may not be gluten free this time.

If your child is old enough, encourage them to practice placing an order themselves, and discussing the need for a gluten free meal. One day (surprisingly soon) they will need to be able to do this without you, and practicing with you there as backup will help.

If you are eating abroad, consider taking a translation card with you. These cards explain the coeliac diet in various languages, and you can buy or download these in the language you need from the internet (Coeliac UK has a good variety).

If your visit goes well, thank the staff and leave a positive review (commenting on the fact that you needed a gluten free meal) on sites such as TripAdvisor or

Facebook. Not only will this help the restaurant out, and encourage them to go on providing gluten free food options, it will make the staff feel good and help future coeliac visitors decide whether to eat there or not.

What should you say to restaurant staff?

It is important that food preparation and serving staff understand that your child has coeliac disease, and that this is a serious condition.

Luckily, understanding of the gluten free diet is improving a great deal here in the UK—though not always helped by people who pick and choose to be gluten free when they want to be. People who say they have to be gluten free at the beginning of the meal but are happy to choose a gluten-full dessert make restaurant staff cynical about the next person in who wants to be gluten free.

This isn't surprising; preparation of a gluten free meal in a mixed gluten-free/gluten-full kitchen will necessitate a lot of extra work for the staff in cleaning down a preparation area to avoid contamination.

However, we know that your child is coeliac, so it is essential that you can make their needs clear. They are relying on you to keep them safe.

Ask for the gluten free menu; you'll be surprised how often there is one. And if there isn't a specific menu, the general menu may be marked up to show what is gluten free. Or there may be a binder of information held by the front of house staff to indicate which dishes contain which allergens.

We used to say something like: "my daughter has coeliac disease, and will be ill if she eats food made with wheat, barley, oats or rye. Is this [whatever it is] OK for her to eat?" These days she's more than capable of dealing with it herself.

Be prepared to discuss any dish that seems appropriate, and to ask for it to be made and presented without bread, croutons, gravy or other gluten-full accompaniment.

If a meal for your coeliac arrives at the table and you are not fully confident that it is OK, you must check. If it arrives with gluten-full accompaniments (croutons are my bugbear: how often do people toss croutons onto salad without thinking about it?) you must send it back and ask for a fresh one; it is definitely not OK for the staff simply to pick off the croutons and re-present it.

Travelling

Be prepared

Always plan ahead and pack a variety of snacks. More snacks than you think your child could possibly eat... delays are always a risk, and will be harder to manage (and to keep your sanity) if you have a hungry child.

I know I already warned you to plan ahead, but travelling with a coeliac child can be made more problematic by difficulties in finding suitable food while on the move. Our coeliac daughter has had many bizarre combinations of foods in an attempt to find enough food to keep her going! And children often can't wait long for a meal once they're hungry.

Travel as a coeliac is getting a lot easier. Here in the UK, gluten free options are becoming very widely available, and we have successfully taken our coeliac daughter to the USA, Egypt, France, Italy, Greece and Spain. And now she's a young adult, she has travelled with friends to Germany, Denmark and Sri Lanka.

So you see, it can be done, though your child may find that they eat a lot of bananas (the coeliac's friend).

Self-catering holidays

We've always preferred to self-cater, because it means that we have control over what food we can offer our coeliac. This does mean that we take an initial set of gluten free supplies with us, for the first few days, and then explore the local supermarkets to see what is available. We've made some interesting finds over the years; for example, when we visited the USA, we came back with several packets of a kind of pasta that she'd particularly enjoyed, and French supermarkets carry biscuits that we just can't buy here in the UK.

Hotels/cruises/tours/airlines

I strongly recommend contacting any organisation that you are expecting to provide your child with food (especially airlines) to let them know about your child's dietary needs. If you're going on a long-haul flight, order a gluten free meal in advance, and then ask at check-in whether it has been arranged. Our experience has been quite poor with some airlines, where a gluten free meal has been ordered, and then it doesn't appear on the plane. Travelling with a hungry child on a long flight is no fun at all, so always take your own supplies as a backup.

Local country guides

The national coeliac organisation in the countries you want to visit may well be able to help with lists of gluten free foods in their country, and maybe with lists of shops/restaurants/hotels that can provide for a gluten free diet.

Don't forget to buy (or maybe download from your national coeliac organisation) translation cards and other information in the language of the countries you want to visit. This can make communication of dietary needs easier when you don't speak the local language.

What about travel insurance?

We have always told our insurers about our daughter's coeliac disease, and haven't had to pay extra. After all, as long as your child sticks to a gluten free diet, they will be as healthy as any other child. If you are charged more because of your child's coeliac disease, then shop around for another quote.

Picky eating

Some children just are picky about what they will or won't eat. And it is very hard to persuade a picky eater to eat. You can't make someone eat; and putting pressure on could cause food issues. But it is very difficult, if you've invested time and money in providing good food for your child, to have them reject it—it can feel as though you've failed in some way.

But it is important that you try not to react; don't season the meal with your own emotions, because this will only make the not-eating into a bigger issue, and make your child more likely to resist.

Stay calm.

No child will starve if food is made available to them. I know this is hard to believe when the health professionals tell you this, as your child refuses to eat your lovingly prepared food yet again. But it is true.

Why is my child being picky?

It may be that your picky eater is picky about food because of coeliac disease. Our daughter gradually reduced the range of foods she would eat before diagnosis to a minimum, but picky eating can manifest before or after diagnosis:

- If they have become malnourished, and aren't getting enough of certain vitamins or minerals, they can look like picky eaters
- If they've made a connection between eating food and experiencing pain and discomfort, that could have led to reluctance to eat
- Intolerances to a food can make someone crave that food, too—so if your child will only eat gluten-full food, it may be the gluten that is causing the problem
- It is possible that your child is anxious about trying new and different foods because they are worried it will make them ill.

So how do you persuade a picky eater to eat gluten free?

Don't go gradually; you do need to remove gluten from their diet completely, so that they can start to heal.

Try preparing only naturally gluten free foods (such as rice, plain meat or fish, yoghurt and fruit) that your picky eater likes, for a while.

The gluten free versions of their favourite things (e.g. bread, chicken nuggets) do taste different, so if you can avoid those things for a while, and then reintroduce them in a gluten free form in a couple of weeks, they may not notice the difference.

Try giving them control over what they choose to eat; within a gluten free selection, of course. For a toddler, for instance, you could put a tiny amount of a variety of foods on a plate, and let them pick and choose.

Don't offer lots of snacks and drinks, so that your child is genuinely hungry at mealtimes.

And if they refuse to eat, just remove the food. They will accept something to eat eventually—just don't offer gluten-full options. If this becomes a real problem, you may have to remove all gluten-full food from the house, so that their only option is to eat gluten free. And be persistent; it may take multiple attempts before your child will accept a new food.

If your picky eater is old enough, you may be able to explain it to them in a way that makes switching to the gluten free diet an interesting challenge, especially if you do it together. Look for books or websites that help them understand coeliac disease and the gluten free diet.

Teens may be interested in helping you research different choices, or choosing menu plans. For pre-teens, sticker-charts and small rewards may help. Taking the child to the supermarket to help you choose might help too.

Try a wide variety of options; some gluten free breads, for instance, are much better than others. You can find gluten free foods to sample for free at food fairs and (often) at your local support group. Some big manufacturers also offer free sample packs, in the hope that you will become a regular customer.

We make a point of going to allergy food fairs so we can see what is new, and try a wide range of things. This can help your child see being gluten free as being special, rather than a problem, as well as exposing them to a variety of different products, and helping them see that they are not the only one.

And if your child was aware of, and distressed by, their symptoms before diagnosis, then they will probably be keen to try anything that will help to make them better.

Be patient; you'll get there. And if you're struggling, talk to your doctor or dietician.

Making mistakes

There will be mistakes

It took us years to make our first one, but inevitably, it happened. We had chips from somewhere we'd had them from before... and didn't check. It turned out that they'd changed their supplier, and now the chips were coated in wheat flour to make them crispy when fried. Our coeliac daughter paid the penalty for our mistake with 24 hours of severe abdominal pain, fever and chills, fainting, vomiting and diarrhoea.

There may be cheating—by the child

I suspect that the younger the child when diagnosed, the less deliberate cheating there'll be; if you don't know what you're missing, and you can't remember any other way of eating, then there'll be less temptation to have something bad 'just this once'.

And the diet is difficult for teenagers in particular, as it is restricting, and creates a significant loss of spontaneity. If the crowd is heading to a particular place for lunch, and there's nothing you can eat on the menu except for corn on the cob, it can be difficult to suggest going somewhere else, and hard not to eat the tempting food that others are eating.

Encourage your child to remember that even if they don't feel any ill effects from eating gluten, it is damaging them on the inside.

There may be deliberate breaches of the diet rules—by other carers

If a relative or other carer doesn't really understand the need for the diet, they may be inclined to offer inappropriate food on the grounds that (for example):

- "just a bit won't matter" (it will)
- "but he loves my cooking, especially my chocolate cake" (yes, but please make it gluten free)
- "that's just a faddy diet, he needs feeding up" (it's a medical necessity)
- "we've always done it this way, and you've all grown up just fine" (but we didn't have coeliac disease)
- Or even: "here's a biscuit, don't tell your mother".
- And, of course, if your child has recovered from their symptoms (by eating gluten free) and therefore doesn't look ill, it can be hard for some people to recognise that they are at risk.

This is obviously going to need careful handling, but don't risk your child's health in the interests of being polite.

You can try:

- Providing informative articles and/or your own fact-sheet
- Explaining (again) what the risks to your child's health are
- Bringing your own food
- Be the cook, if you can.

Explain to your child (when they are old enough) that some people don't know that they have coeliac disease or just don't understand how bad gluten is for them.

Ignore the comments if you can; just focus on keeping your child healthy. And if relatives won't pay any attention to your child's needs, do you really have to eat with them?

What treatment to provide if there is a mistake?

First of all, don't panic. It is very, very unlikely to be life-threatening.

Symptoms shown by one child before diagnosis may well have been different to those shown by another child. Similarly, the symptoms they show if there is a mistake may vary. Indeed, a child may have shown one set of symptoms before diagnosis, and show different symptoms if there is a mistake.

The most likely symptoms, though, include cramps, diarrhoea, vomiting, severe fatigue, headache and brain fog (inability to concentrate). Symptoms could appear within a few hours or in a day or so, and could take a few hours or a few days to disappear.

But there is little by way of medication that you can offer that will help. Rest, rehydration and a simple light diet when they feel ready to eat again will all help. You can buy flavoured rehydration sachets from your pharmacist, or you can make your own with clean boiled water, sugar and salt (search online for a recipe). Or flat coke works well; just pour coke in a glass and stir for a while to release the bubbles.

If your child is older, they might find that peppermint tea or ginger tea helps.

Is your child struggling with temptation? Try this

Don't be tempted by people who suggest that *"a little bit won't hurt"*, urge *"just this once"*, or say *"go on—I won't tell anybody"*, while offering you a plate of gluten-full food.

Your health is worth more than the moment's pleasure that a proper croissant might give. Yes it is! Even if you don't suffer any symptoms in the next few days, you will have done yourself some internal damage, and it will take much longer for that damage to heal than it did for you to eat that tempting treat.

Not only that, but you might feel less good about yourself. Are you really the sort of person who can't say no? And if you give in this time, you are setting yourself up to be tempted by these people again, as they won't understand that gluten free is for life if you don't explain it to them clearly enough.

So—health, self-esteem and an easier life? I'd say you were worth it!

Avoid negativity

Is your child's packed lunch safe?

I once read a message from a parent whose daughter is coeliac. One of the other children at school had taken to 'accidentally' dropping not-gluten-free food into her packed lunch, rendering it inedible.

I think this is classic bullying. It's important that any school understands the serious effect this could have.

If the child throws her food away because she knows it is contaminated, then she'll be hungry, and not able to concentrate

If the child gambles, and eats the food, she could suffer:

- Vomiting and/or diarrhoea (neither of which the teacher will enjoy having to deal with in class)
- Brain fog, making her unable to concentrate
- And possibly a host of other symptoms, as well as long-term damage.

This is obviously bad for the child, but also difficult for the teachers and other staff.

Luckily we've never had to handle this kind of bullying. We've had to deal with other bullying (both physical and psychological), but never anything to do with being gluten free.

If your child is experiencing anything like this, start with a request for a meeting with the teacher, and if that doesn't help, escalate to the head teacher. And a letter from your doctor to the head outlining the medical risks would get their attention.

It's just good manners

Every family has its own traditions and in-jokes. One of ours is Rule 17b.

When my children were little, and we were trying to teach them acceptable table manners, the number of rules about what they should/shouldn't do at the table seemed to get ever longer.

Rule 17b came about as a joke rule—something to do with not-deliberately-humming-in-a-way-that-annoys-your-sister-at-the-table—and is now used as a general hint about behaviour.

One of the rules that my sister has is that no-one should be rude about anyone else's food. As an experienced foster-mother, she's dealt with a lot of children with a variety of food-related and behavioural issues, and I was impressed by this rule when I first heard her invoke it.

I wished I could have used it a while ago. My coeliac daughter—then a Young Leader at Guides—was eating, picnic style, with her group of Guides, and one of them commented on her food:

"Oh yes, I used to have to eat gluten-free. It's disgusting, isn't it?"

Hmm. My daughter has a core of steel, and wasn't affected—but someone younger, more recently diagnosed, or struggling with the diet might have found this kind of comment very hard to deal with. Especially from someone who presumably has experienced the difficulties of a special diet—and who was certainly old enough to know better.

Definitely a call for Rule 17b, which may need to be rewritten:

"No-one should be rude about anyone else's food."

And yes, that includes your child, who shouldn't be rude about gluten-full food either.

Teach your child how to refuse food politely

Inevitably, your child will be offered food that they can't eat at some point. They'll need strategies for dealing with this, and they'll need to practice.

Sometimes, a simple *"no thank you"* will be enough. But they will need to be able to explain the problem if they are pressed.

"Thank you, but I have coeliac disease and will be ill if I eat gluten"

"That looks delicious, but I don't know if I can eat it. Is there any wheat, barley or rye in it?"

"I have coeliac disease and must be careful what I eat or I will be ill. Please could I look at the packet to read the ingredients?"

Teach your child to cook

Teach your child to cook; and if you don't know how, learn together.

A coeliac who can cook from scratch will be able to prepare healthy meals that they know are gluten free, and which are likely to be cheaper than the ready-made gluten free meals available in the supermarkets.

Once your child has mastered a few basic skills, they can be combined into a variety of different meals.

Depending on the age of your child, I'd suggest starting with baking, because every child enjoys mixing up ingredients and eating the results. But children can cook (with supervision) from very young.

We made sure that our coeliac had a small repertoire of meals requiring different skills before she left to go to university (where she cooks for herself). The skills included how to:

- chop a variety of vegetables (e.g. onions and garlic as ingredients, potatoes and other vegetables for hot meal accompaniments, salad vegetables to make a salad)
- beat eggs (scrambled eggs, omelettes, baking)
- Separate egg white from egg yolks, and whisk the egg whites (meringues, souffles)
- make a white sauce (which can become a cheese sauce by adding grated cheese)
- make a tomato-based sauce (which can be the basis for another dish, or served with pasta)
- cook mince (to make chilli, bolognese, lasagne etc)
- brown chunks of meat on the cooker top (to go into other dishes)
- oven-cook chicken breasts and fish fillets (which could be served with a cheese sauce, or with a tomato sauce)
- coat chicken breasts and fish with egg and gluten free breadcrumbs or other coatings, such as gluten free cornflakes or crisps (to make, for instance, gluten free fish fingers)

- make risotto—once you've understood the technique, you can add a range of ingredients to create different flavours
- make fishcakes—once you've understood the principle of binding ingredients into small patties, you can make a variety of different things
- bake cookies and chocolate brownie.

Once the skills are mastered, the range of dishes that use these skills is wide, and, perhaps more importantly, your child will have the confidence to try learning new skills and experimenting with new recipes.

For example, once you can make a gluten free white sauce, you can add flavourings to it (usually cheese in our house, but herbs work well). And with a cheese sauce (and maybe a few additional skills from the list above), you know how to make:

- macaroni cheese
- cauliflower cheese
- fish pie
- pasta bake
- lasagne
- moussaka
- gratin (with leeks and/or potatoes or other vegetables)
- souffle
- cream soups
- sauce for eggs/fish/meat/vegetables/croquettes /fishcakes... (e.g. add spinach for eggs florentine)
- and lots more.

Adapting recipes to be gluten free can be very easy. For example, consider using crushed gluten free crisps (chips, if you're American) or rice krispie cereal as a coating for chicken or fish instead of breadcrumbs. For a while, when the children were younger, our homemade gluten free chicken nuggets and fish fingers were preferred by our non-coeliac children to the shop-bought version.

It is important for your child to enjoy eating, and if they also enjoy cooking, they are likely to be able to provide themselves with a healthy diet for the rest of their lives. And that is something that everyone, whether they have coeliac disease or not, should be able to do.

Coeliac disease and the gluten free diet

Common symptoms

There are over 200 different signs and symptoms of the disease, though some people who show no symptoms at all can still have coeliac disease.

This means that it can sometimes be misdiagnosed as something else (irritable bowel syndrome, for example), though the diagnosis rate is improving as people become more aware of it. If you think this could be the case, then you should go back to your doctor to discuss the symptoms.

Common symptoms include:

- Anaemia
- Brain fog
- Constipation
- Cramps (abdominal pain)
- Diarrhoea
- Fatigue
- Failure to thrive (in infants—not keeping up with the growth charts)
- Foul-smelling stools
- Malnutrition (looks like: distended stomach, skinny arms, legs and buttocks)
- Mouth ulcers
- Pale stools
- Vomiting
- Vitamin deficiency
- Weight change (loss or gain)

It is very unlikely that your child had all of these symptoms, and as we said above, it is possible to have silent coeliac disease in which no symptoms are shown.

Our daughter suffered from vomiting and diarrhoea, pale, foul-smelling stools, malnutrition and failure to thrive. She also lacked energy to move about and play. It took us some months to get to a final diagnosis, and we were lucky to have an experienced GP who suspected it from the start. For some people, diagnosis can take years. This is improving as awareness increases.

Other symptoms or potentially related conditions include:

- ADHD
- Anxiety
- Arthritis
- Ataxia / clumsiness
- Bloating
- Delayed puberty
- Dental enamel defects
- Depression
- Diabetes
- Down syndrome
- Heartburn
- Infertility
- Irritable bowel syndrome
- Itchy skin rash (Dermatitis Herpetiformis)
- Joint pain
- Lactose intolerance
- Lupus
- Numbness or tingling in hands or feet

- Miscarriage
- Osteopenia / Osteoporosis
- Rheumatoid arthritis
- Psoriasis
- Rheumatoid arthritis
- Sjogren syndrome
- Thyroid disease
- Turner syndrome

There are many, many more.

Steps to diagnosis

If your child is showing symptoms of coeliac disease then discuss them with a doctor. Don't remove gluten from your child's diet yet.

Likely first step: blood tests

The first test for coeliac disease is usually a blood test. This blood test is looking for antibodies that the body makes in response to eating gluten, and is looking for IgA (Total immunoglobulin A) and IgA tTG (tissue transglutaminase). If the IgA tTG test is weakly positive, then IgA EMA (endomysial antibodies) should be used.

This will give the doctors some indication of whether it is coeliac disease or not. However, this test can be wrong: it is possible to have a negative test, but still have coeliac disease.

Usually, here in the UK at least, your child will be given some 'magic cream' or 'magic spray' before the blood is taken. This is a simple local anaesthetic. In our experience, waiting for the magic cream to work before having the blood test taken is worse than the blood test itself. Go for the spray if you can, especially if your child is young or particularly anxious—it works instantly, and this cuts down the wait time, during which the worry builds up.

Possible second step: biopsy

If the blood test is positive, or if there is still suspicion of coeliac disease even after a negative test, then the next step could be a biopsy. This will involve passing a thin flexible tube with a tiny camera down through the mouth into the small intestine, where small samples of the gut lining will be collected for examination.

Although this is the traditional gold standard diagnosis tool for coeliac disease, it does have its limitations. Some areas of the intestine may still look healthy, while others may be very damaged, so it is advised to take five or six samples from different parts of the intestine. These samples are then sent to a pathology lab where pathologists look for signs of coeliac disease.

The biopsy itself doesn't hurt, but it is important that the patient stays still. So in young children, this test is done under anaesthetic—or at least sedation, which is what my daughter had (liquid on a spoon).

Don't be alarmed if there's a lot of interest in this procedure; student doctors don't often get to see such a test, so there will be a surprising number of people present.

Be aware that if your child is sedated rather than anaesthetised, they may still struggle against swallowing the tube. This isn't pleasant, but they won't remember.

Also, be prepared to be excluded from the procedure at some point. We weren't warned of this, but although I was allowed to go with her to the door, I wasn't allowed to accompany her in for the test. She was returned minutes later when she was waking up (and retching from having the tube removed). And then she got up to move about, as toddlers do, but looked like a small drunkard, staggering about woozily. We weren't allowed to leave until she'd eaten something.

Don't stop feeding your child gluten until the biopsy is complete, because the results will be inaccurate; their intestines will start to heal, and the villi to regrow.

Do we really need to do a biopsy?

If the blood tests are very clear, your medical team may decide not to conduct a biopsy (it is, after all, invasive, and does require sedation).

The guidance at the moment (from the European Society for Paediatric Gastroenterology Hepatology and Nutrition 2012) is that if a child shows 10 times the normal anti-TTG, then a second test (this time for IgA endomysial antibodies—EMA) could be conducted, and if that were also positive, the child could go gluten free. If, then, the child's antibodies returned to normal, coeliac disease could be considered to be proven.

So some specialists believe that the biopsy is no longer necessarily the gold standard for diagnosis, though this is controversial. Here in the UK, for instance, in Derby, about half of coeliac patients are diagnosed using blood tests alone.

However, there is some concern in the US that patients diagnosed by blood test alone tend to be less compliant with the gluten free diet over time than those who have seen an image of the damage caused by gluten to their intestine. That is because if you could see the damage that gluten is doing to the gut, there'd be no temptation to cheat.

If your child's medical professionals advise that your child should have a biopsy, it is up to you whether or not to accept that advice. I'd just say that our experience of the biopsy was that it was nothing to worry about and it was worth getting the confirmation that she does, indeed, have coeliac disease.

What about genetic testing?

Coeliac disease is, after all, a genetic disease, so what can be done by genetic testing?

Genetic testing can determine whether someone has a high or a low risk for coeliac disease, but is really only used to 'rule out' coeliac disease. Someone who tests negative for the coeliac disease genetic markers is unlikely to have coeliac disease, so wouldn't need monitoring (for example, testing the child of a coeliac parent would indicate whether that child had inherited the propensity to develop coeliac disease). Or, for example, if someone had been on a gluten free diet because they'd shown symptoms of coeliac disease, but hadn't had a biopsy, then a negative gene test would indicate that those symptoms were not due to coeliac disease.

Still not feeling better?

I hope that after a very few weeks on the gluten free diet, your child begins to feel better. It can take longer for all the symptoms to clear up completely.

However, in some cases, people diagnosed with coeliac disease still have symptoms even once they've been on a gluten free diet for a while (6-12 months).

There are a number of possible reasons for this:
- Incorrect diagnosis of coeliac disease
- Gluten is still in the diet somewhere
- Lactose intolerance
- Non-coeliac gluten sensitivity
- Irritable bowel syndrome
- Some other condition exists in addition to coeliac disease
- Refractory coeliac disease.

Incorrect diagnosis of coeliac disease

This is unusual, but worth discussing with your doctor if your child hasn't had a biopsy, or if the pathology review of the biopsy was inconclusive for coeliac disease for any reason—there are other causes of blunted villi, but most of these other conditions can be excluded.

A gluten challenge used to be standard procedure, to check the diagnosis; this is very rare these days, and it shouldn't be necessary if a biopsy has been performed. A challenge is a period of time during which gluten is eaten again (which could be as long as six weeks) to see if symptoms recur, followed by repeat testing.

Twenty years ago, when our daughter was first diagnosed, we were told that she'd have to go through a gluten challenge when she was a bit older to confirm whether or not she was a coeliac. This would be done by sprinkling gluten in the form of a powder onto her food. A few years later, this was no longer standard procedure, so we've never had to put her through a challenge, and it's likely that you won't have to do that either.

Hidden gluten

This is the most likely cause of continued symptoms.

It may be that your child is still eating gluten somehow. Gluten is in all sorts of different things, and it is easy to miss something: you'll need to check absolutely everything that they are eating (including play items such as play-dough and glue).

It may be helpful to see a dietician, for advice on hidden gluten. If you haven't already, join your local support group, who may also have some good ideas about where gluten may be lurking.

It could be as simple as using the same spoon to stir gluten free food as you've just used to stir not-gluten-free food (see the contamination section).

Lactose intolerance

Newly diagnosed with coeliac disease, cut out gluten completely, but still having trouble digesting dairy products? Your child could be suffering from secondary lactose intolerance.

Lactose intolerance can have a genetic cause:

- Congenital: the ability to digest lactose could have been absent from birth
- Developmental: the ability to digest lactose could have diminished over time.

Or lactose intolerance could be caused by a disease that damages the lining of the small intestine—such as coeliac disease. This is called secondary lactose intolerance.

Eating gluten causes an immune reaction which shortens, or even flattens, the villi, resulting in a decrease in the digestive enzymes—and these enzymes include lactase, which helps digest the lactose found in milk. If you don't have enough lactase, you can't digest lactose, resulting in those all too familiar symptoms of nausea, diarrhoea, stomach pain and bloating.

Once you've stopped eating gluten, and the gut starts to heal, the villi—and microvilli—will regenerate. For most people with secondary lactose intolerance, this will mean that they can digest milk products again. It often takes six months to a year, and can take two years.

(Be aware that lactose intolerance is not the same as a milk allergy.)

Secondary lactose intolerance: treatment

Assuming that it is lactose intolerance, what should you do while you're waiting for your child's villi to regenerate?

Lactose is found in milk from cows, sheep and goats, so cutting out these milks is an obvious response.

But people vary: some may be able to have a small amount of milk, while others find even a small amount triggers symptoms.

And don't just cut out lactose completely without consulting your GP or dietitian for advice, because your child may miss out on other essential nutrients, such as calcium, potassium, magnesium, zinc, and vitamins A, B12 and D.

In addition, there does seem to be evidence that people can eat some cheese (but not milk) even if they are lactose intolerant. Studies show that many people can tolerate a small amount (10-12g) of lactose daily—and the amount of lactose in milk / yoghurt and cheese varies:

- 6 ounces of low fat plain yoghurt contains 13g lactose
- 6 ounces of low fat Greek yoghurt contains 4g lactose
- ½ cup of low fat cottage cheese contains 3g lactose
- 1 ounce of cheddar cheese or other hard cheese contains under 1g lactose.

Try (a small amount to start with of) hard cheese such as cheddar or gruyere. The reason for choosing hard cheese is that in the cheese-making process, starter cultures of bacteria are added to milk that turns lactose into lactic acid. Starter cultures are usually used to make aged cheeses, not fresh ones.

Dieticians also suggest eating yoghurt, hard cheese or a small amount of milk as part of a meal, rather than on its own, because that will help.

But be aware that milk products appear in all sorts of other foods, so your child might get up to the limit that they can tolerate without even realising it. So always check the label. (Just like looking for gluten, really).

In the EU, manufactured foods will clearly list if milk or an ingredient derived from milk is contained in the product. But if you are not in the EU, you will need to look out for:

- Milk powder / skimmed milk powder
- Milk drinks / malted milk drinks (malted milk is not gluten free, in any case)
- Cheese / cheese powder
- Butter
- Margarine or other low fat spread (unless it says it is dairy free)
- Yoghurt / fromage frais
- Cream / sour cream
- Casein / caseinates / sodium caseinates / hydrolysed casein
- Milk solids
- Non-fat milk
- Whey / Whey syrup sweetener
- Milk sugar solids
- and, obviously, lactose.

For some people who are intolerant to cows milk, it appears that it is one of the proteins in cows milk—A1 casein—that is causing the problem, rather than lactose. Although there are some breeds of cow that don't produce A1 casein—and A2 milk can be bought as a specialist product in most supermarkets here in the UK these days—most cows used in standard mass dairy production are A1 producers. (Note: both A1 milk and A2 milk contain lactose, so A2 milk is not an option if your child is lactose intolerant or has a milk allergy).

Goats milk contains only A2 casein, which means that for some people, goats milk is much less inflammatory than cows milk—so if you're trying to avoid the A1 casein, goats milk products are a good choice.

And although goats milk contains lactose, it seems some people with lactose intolerance can handle goats milk. It is thought that this may be because goats milk is more digestible—it has less casein, smaller fat globules, and very slightly less lactose, than cows milk.

And if that's not enough, it turns out that goats milk is very high in potassium and calcium, as well as tryptophan—so it works very well to help people with sleeping problems.

Non-coeliac gluten sensitivity

About 1 in 100 people have coeliac disease. For most of the rest of the population, there is no reason to avoid gluten. But for some, coeliac-type symptoms exist, but they do not have the coeliac disease antibodies, and a biopsy doesn't reveal damage to the lining of the intestine.

So what is going on?

Theories vary. It may be the placebo effect (people expect to feel better on a gluten free diet and so they do); it may be that they are in the early stages of coeliac disease, and aren't showing any symptoms yet; it may be that they are allergic to wheat; or it may be that they are sensitive to FODMAPs (certain carbohydrates, including the carbohydrates in wheat, lentils and mushrooms).

This kind of problem has been named non-coeliac gluten sensitivity (NCGS). There isn't yet a reliable diagnosis test, and the symptoms can vary—like the symptoms of coeliac disease.

The first thing to do is to go back to the doctor to discuss the symptoms, and—assuming that coeliac disease has been ruled out—to discuss the possibility of non coeliac gluten sensitivity.

Irritable bowel syndrome and FODMAPs

Coeliac disease and irritable bowel syndrome (IBS) have a lot in common—both can cause diarrhoea, constipation, cramps and so on—but there are key differences.

Coeliac disease is an autoimmune disorder that damages the lining of the small intestine; in IBS the intestines do not follow the regular movement pattern of a 'normal' body, and this constant squeezing causes discomfort. Coeliac disease can have a wide range of non-gastrointestinal symptoms; IBS does not.

Because of the potential for confusion, studies have found that around 16% of people with coeliac disease are first misdiagnosed as having IBS. Delay in diagnosis leads to further intestinal damage, which can lead to secondary related conditions such as anaemia. It is important to get a correct diagnosis because the treatment is different. So if your child has been diagnosed with IBS, but you suspect it could be coeliac disease, do discuss it with your doctor.

It is possible to have both, so if your child has already been diagnosed with coeliac disease but is still having symptoms, do discuss it with your doctor.

It is possible that a low FODMAP diet would help reduce continuing symptoms. FODMAPs are fermentable oligosaccharides, disaccharides, monosaccharides and polyols (no wonder people shorten this to FODMAP), and the low FODMAP diet was developed in 1999 in Australia to control symptoms associated with IBS. Because foods high in FODMAPs may not be easy to digest, they can ferment in the large intestine, causing gas, bloating, cramps, nausea and changes in bowel function.

Wheat, barley and rye, which contain gluten, as we know, are also high in FODMAPs, so the gluten free diet would reduce the FODMAPs in the diet, but not eliminate them. You'd need to remove some other high FODMAP foods as well.

The FODMAP diet is beyond the scope of this ebook, and you should discuss it with a doctor and a dietician.

Another condition exists

It is of course entirely possible to have two similar health problems at the same time. If symptoms continue, then it may be worth considering whether some other condition exists as well. There are several potential candidates, including Crohn's disease, giardia, microscopic colitis, pancreatic insufficiency or inflammatory bowel disease.

Refractory coeliac disease

In refractory coeliac disease, the lining of the intestine does not heal on a gluten free diet.

This is very rare, and when it is found, it is typically in older people (over 50) newly diagnosed with coeliac disease, so your child is not likely to be affected by this.

Talk to your doctor, who will recommend further tests as well as discussions with a dietician, and, if things don't improve, appropriate treatment.

It is essential that your child sticks to the gluten free diet even if they are still having symptoms to avoid future complications.

What can your child eat?

You finally got a diagnosis for your child, and they said "Don't eat anything containing wheat, oats, barley or rye—avoid all gluten".

OK—but what does that mean? What can your child eat?

Your first thought might be "oh, that's not so bad—only four things to avoid" but after a trip to the supermarket, and looking at some labels, you might be thinking "They're going to starve".

Luckily, the truth is in-between, and you may both end up with a healthier diet than when they were eating gluten, because you'll probably eat more fresh and home-prepared food together.

Do try to eat as a family, sharing the same meal, whenever you can; sharing food is an important part of social bonding, and will matter throughout your child's life: at school, at work, and at social events. All children need to practice this skill, and it is just that bit harder for the coeliac, who may already feel different without having it highlighted at every meal.

So—what can we eat?

The good news is that there are a lot of different things that are gluten free and safe to eat:

- Cereals and grains: rice, millet, maize, quinoa, tapioca, sago, buckwheat, teff and sorghum
- Meat fish, and eggs: all are basically fine if unprocessed. Just check any coatings, sauces and

spices you add, and check wafer-thin meats too (sometimes wheat flour is added to make them peel apart easily)

- Dairy products: milk and most cream, cheese and yoghurt. Do check any added ingredients, and check ready-grated cheese (sometimes wheat flour is added to stop the slivers of cheese sticking together). Note that blue cheese is regarded as gluten free, despite concerns some people have about the source of the mould that creates the characteristic blue veining
- Flours: rice, corn, potato, maize, gram, soya, chickpea, sorghum, tapioca and chestnut flours are all OK. Obviously, look out for wheat flour, barley flour or rye flour as these are not gluten free (and be wary of oat flour—see the discussion of oats elsewhere in this book)
- Fruit: all fruits are naturally gluten free. Check ready-made pie fillings, though, in case they've been thickened with flour
- Vegetables: all vegetables are naturally gluten free. Check any coatings, sauces and spices, and check whether potato chips (fries) have been dusted in wheat flour or fried in oil used to fry gluten-containing foods.
- Fats: butter, margarine, oils, lard and dripping are all safe to eat, but avoid suet unless you can find a gluten free version (it does exist, but you'll have to look for it) and do check low-fat spreads
- Breakfast cereal: check carefully, and avoid any containing wheat, oats, barley or rye. Also, do avoid

malt extract—some can tolerate this, but most can't (and your child's ability to tolerate it might change over time, too)

- Bread, crackers and crispbreads: avoid all the conventional ones, and eat only those labelled as gluten free, or those you've made yourself and know to be gluten free
- Cakes, pastries, cookies and biscuits: avoid all the conventional ones, and eat only those labelled as gluten free, or those you've made yourself and know to be gluten free
- Pizza and pasta: avoid all the conventional ones, and eat only those labelled as gluten free, or those you've made yourself and know to be gluten free
- Soup and sauces: check every time, in case wheat flour has been used to thicken a soup or a sauce
- Pies, quiches, flans and tarts: avoid all the conventional ones, and eat only those labelled as gluten free, or those you've made yourself and know to be gluten free
- Puddings and desserts: check every time—meringue, jelly and most ice-creams and sorbets will be fine (check the icecream doesn't contain cookies), but unless specifically labelled gluten free, cheesecakes, pies etc will not be safe
- Snacks: nuts, raisins and seeds are all naturally gluten free, but check any added coatings and check all packets of crisps (called chips in America) and other savoury snacks—we've been caught out by these before, especially when the recipe is changed

- Sweets (candy): check every time—chocolate is usually OK to eat, but not if it covers a biscuit! All sorts of unexpected sweets contain wheat, such as Smarties, seaside rock, and licorice. Look for gluten free versions; they do exist
- Alcohol: wine, spirits, liqueurs and cider—avoid real ale, beer, lager and stout (unless specifically labelled as gluten free)
- Soft drinks: coffee, tea, juices, cocoa, fizzy drinks and most squashes—but check that they don't contain barley or 'cloud', and don't drink from vending machines
- Spices and seasonings: pure salt, pepper, and herbs are all gluten free—check spices and mustard powder for added flour
- Vinegar: avoid malt vinegar, but other vinegars should be fine
- Spreads and preserves: jam, marmalade, honey, nut butters should all be naturally gluten free
- Pickles, dressings and other condiments: check every time, because malt vinegar can be included in pickles and soy sauce is rarely gluten free
- Cooking ingredients: yeast, bicarbonate of soda and cream of tartar are OK, but check baking powder for added flour.

There—that's not so bad, is it? Lots to choose from, the range of products available gluten free is expanding all the time, and you'll soon get in the habit of checking food labels and asking for the recipe.

What counts as gluten free?

Many foods are naturally gluten free, but obviously in preparation they can be combined with gluten-containing ingredients—either on purpose, that is, as part of a recipe, or accidentally (when it is usually known as contamination).

The standard by which gluten free foods are measured is in the proportion of gluten to non-gluten-containing ingredients, but the level that this is set to is different in different countries.

A food can be called gluten free (in the UK, Europe, USA, and some others*) if it contains less than 20 parts of gluten per million parts (parts per million = ppm). That is, it doesn't contain enough wheat, barley or rye to trigger symptoms in most coeliac sufferers.

'Most' coeliac sufferers: there are a few for whom 20ppm is too much, but for most people, this extremely low level is acceptable and doesn't cause damage.

*Note: in Australia and New Zealand, there is a zero tolerance rule: that is, levels of gluten must be so low as to be undetectable. Since current technology can measure the level of gluten down to less than 3ppm, this means there is less than 3ppm in gluten free foods in Australia and New Zealand.

What can't your child eat?

We've discussed what your child can eat: what can't they eat?

You already know that wheat, barley and rye are not gluten free. Recent studies indicate that some coeliacs can tolerate contamination-free oats in small portions. It would be sensible to check with your consultant or dietician, and perhaps get fully back to normal before trying oats. We're not giving oats to our daughter—though she's been diagnosed for 20 years.

But labelling is confusing, and those three grains can appear under a variety of different names. Avoid the following ingredients:

- Atta (chapatti flour)
- Barley, barley flakes, barley flour, pearl barley, pot barley, scotch barley
- Bran
- Breadcrumbs (unless labelled gluten free
- Bulgar
- Cereal extract
- Couscous
- Cracked wheat
- Durum wheat
- Einkorn (wheat)
- Emmer (wheat)
- Farina
- Farro / faro
- Flour
- Fu—dried gluten used in some Asian dishes
- Gluten

- Graham flour
- Kamut
- Malt (malt extract, malt syrup, malt flavouring, malt vinegar, malted milk)
- Modified starch (unless it states it is from a 'safe' source, e.g. rice starch or potato starch)
- Matzo, matxo meal
- Oat bran, oats, oatmeal, oat flour
- Porridge oats, rolled oats
- Rusk
- Rye flour
- Seitan (pure gluten)
- Semolina
- Spelt (this is low gluten, but not safe for coeliacs)
- Triticale (a newer grain, a cross between wheat and rye)
- Wheat bran
- Wheat germ
- Wheat flour
- Wheat starch
- Wholemeal flour
- Wholewheat
- Wheat.

Most of these items are rarely seen on ingredients labels. You will quickly get used to what is and what isn't going to be OK to eat. Sausages here in the UK, for instance, almost always contain rusk, which is essentially breadcrumbs (so not good to eat unless they explicitly say gluten free). Burgers sometimes contain rusk too. So some things need careful checking. On the other hand, labelling is getting better, which is making life a lot better.

What about oats?

We were advised, 20 years ago, that our daughter should avoid oats entirely. Later (maybe 10 years ago), the professionals decided that now she was older, she could eat a small amount of gluten free oats daily, and these days, of course, gluten free oats are readily available.

Oats contain soluble and insoluble fibre. The soluble fibre helps to lower cholesterol; the insoluble fibre is good for digestion. Oats also contain important minerals. So oats are good for you. According to studies in Scandinavia, children introduced to oats early in life are less likely to develop persistent asthma, and adding oats to a gluten free diet results in an increased intake of vitamins and minerals as well as fibre.

So what is the issue with oats?

Often, oats are contaminated with wheat, barley and rye in harvesting and processing. So an ordinary packet of oats can't be guaranteed to be free of gluten. Gluten free oats, on the other hand, are grown and processed away from these other grains; so, in theory, they should be safe for most people.

Some people are still sensitive even to uncontaminated oats. Oats contain avenin, which is similar to gluten; most people with coeliac disease can eat avenin, but not everyone.

Note that a pack of 'pure oats' doesn't necessarily mean that they are gluten free, so if you decide to include oats in your child's diet, make sure you use the ones labelled as gluten free.

What else should I know about?

And then there is malt. It comes from barley, and your child should definitely avoid pure malt extract, malt syrup, malt vinegar (unless distilled) malt flour or malted drinks. Malt extract is widely used as a flavouring, especially in breakfast cereals, and is only present in tiny amounts; even so, if you are unsure, avoid it. We do.

What about glucose syrup or maltodextrin?

These ingredients often worry people.

Glucose syrup can be derived from wheat, but because of the production methods, there is no significant gluten in it; it is gluten free.

Maltodextrin is also gluten free. Like glucose syrup, it can be made from wheat, but the production methods mean that it is gluten free. It is not made from barley, even though it sounds like it might be because of the 'malt' at the beginning of the word.

Some people are allergic to wheat; if this is the case, these ingredients may cause problems if they have been made from wheat. Wheat allergy is not the same as coeliac disease, so it is possible, though not usual, to have both at the same time.

It is important to remember that wheat free is not the same as gluten free. Rye bread, for instance, might be wheat free if there is no wheat in it, but not gluten free, because there is gluten in rye.

Some gluten free breads and other products contain wheat with the gluten removed to CODEX Alimentarius standards (i.e. very low amounts remaining—less than 20 parts per million). If your child must be wheat free, you should avoid these CODEX products because they still contain wheat. It is possible, if their symptoms are not disappearing, that they are a sensitive coeliac and should also avoid these CODEX products.

The list of things that are safe to eat is much longer than the list of things to avoid. Unfortunately, the bad things are widespread, and you must check everything until you are used to your child's new diet. And then check some more, because things change:

New! Improved! New Recipe! Now 90% fat-free!

isn't always a good thing.

And what can your child drink?

You know your child can't eat gluten ... but what can you give them to drink?

We're not discussing sugar, or general health here, so do bear that in mind too!

Cold, soft drinks

- Water—whether tap, mineral or flavoured should be fine. There's no gluten in pure water, and we should all be drinking more water
- Pure fruit juice—no gluten in this—just flavour and vitamins (and, sadly, calories from the sugars). Be careful about smoothies—these are usually just fruit juice and yoghurt, but do sometimes have other ingredients, so just check

- Milk is gluten free, though check the ingredients in milk shakes. If your child is lactose intolerant, or avoiding dairy for other reasons, try soya milk or rice milk. You may find your child can manage goat's milk
- Most fizzy drinks are gluten free (though check for malt extract) but be careful about cloudy fizzy drinks, which can contain wheat starch in the 'cloud', which is added to improve the appearance of the drink
- Most fruit squashes are gluten free, but don't drink the 'fruit and barley' squashes. It would seem obvious, but you'd be surprised how easy it is to miss this!
- Probiotic drinks are a new trend. Check them, but they should be fine if you can handle dairy products.

Hot drinks

- Plain tea is gluten free, as should be any milk or sugar that you add, but be wary of drinks from vending machines, as there may be cross-contamination
- Herbal or fruit teas and infusions that you make with a bag should all be gluten free (though be wary, as sometimes the bag may be sealed with glue containing gluten)
- Plain coffee is gluten free (and so are milk and sugar, though be careful about shared sugar bowls, in case of double-dipping) but be careful of flavourings and other additions (e.g. some chocolate toppings to go on cappuccinos, lattes, etc). Again, be careful about using vending machines

- Coffee substitutes, such as chicory blends or decaffeinated drinks may contain gluten
- Pure instant chicory is gluten free
- Chocolate drinks: pure cocoa powder is gluten free, but check drinking chocolate because this can contain wheat
- Savoury drinks, such as Bovril should be checked carefully
- Avoid malted drinks (because of the malt). Malt extract and malt flavouring are made from barley, and widely used in breakfast cereals, pre-prepared meals, sweets and snacks. Small amounts of malt extract can be tolerated by many coeliacs, but not everyone, so check, and be careful. Even if your child can handle a bowl of cereal, they may tip themselves over the 'safe' limit if they eat malt repeatedly throughout the day.

And what about my teenage child, or young adult?

- Cider, sherry, port and liqueurs are gluten free. Some fortified wines and sherry may contain caramel colour, which may be derived from wheat starch, but which doesn't contain detectable gluten, and is considered to be gluten free
- Wine should be gluten free, whether still, fizzy, sweet or dry, but we have had reports that some wines are treated with hydrolysed wheat gluten as part of the fining process. Again, the level of gluten is not

detectable in the final product, and it is considered to be gluten free

- Spirits are gluten free as long as no gluten product is added after distillation. Yes, including malt whiskies, because of the distillation process. But be careful of cocktails, which may have a gluten-containing product in them, depending on the recipe
- Most beer, lager, stout and ale contain gluten, so avoid these. There are a growing range of gluten free beers of all varieties available.

Reading the label

Of course, nothing is ever quite that easy.

Gluten is hidden in some quite unexpected places. I can't say it too often: always read the label.

Here in the UK, if a recipe for a product includes wheat, barley, rye (or oats), then that ingredient must be written in bold in the ingredients list. This has made reading labels much easier than it used to be. However, the law doesn't cover accidental contamination of ingredients with gluten-containing ingredients.

May contain gluten

You will see pack labels on food that say "may contain gluten". This is known as precautionary allergen labelling.

This is confusing, and can be worrying. Does it mean that the product probably does contain gluten or probably doesn't? Is it just legal-speak, covering the manufacturers in case something sneaks in? Is it safe to eat?

And if there isn't a "may contain" label, does that mean it is safe to eat, or that the manufacturer just hasn't put it on the label?

The result of this confusion is that either you have to decide to ignore these warnings, or to reduce the variety of foods available to your child by paying attention to the warnings. Only you can make that choice, I'm afraid.

If it helps, we tend to ignore the precautionary allergen labels based on our level of trust of the manufacturer, and haven't had a problem as a result. But everyone is different, and your attitude to the risk may vary depending on how sensitive you or your child is to gluten.

There is a campaign running to try to develop an independent accreditation system, so that consumers can feel reassured about the safety of their food choices. It hasn't been set up yet, but keep an eye out for news on this front.

Wheat free is not the same as gluten free

You'll remember that gluten is found in barley and rye as well as in wheat. Wheat seems to get all the publicity, probably because it is more common in our diets. But barley and rye will also affect your child, so don't assume that just because something is wheat free it is also free from barley or rye.

What do I feed my baby?

Perhaps it's you that has coeliac disease, and you're worried about your new baby?

As we've said, if you have coeliac disease, there is an increased risk that your baby could also develop it, and if you're expecting a baby, or have a newborn, you're probably worrying about this.

While ideally you'd probably prefer your child not to have this condition, there are good reasons not to worry:

- Because you know that there is an increased risk, you'll be able to watch out for potential symptoms, and get them tested early if it looks like they may have developed the condition. This could save your child months of illness, pain, missed growth and other issues. If only we'd known our daughter was at risk...

- You have the experience to help them stay safe and healthy if they do have it. Though parents without prior experience of the gluten free diet learn fast, as we had to!

- And if they have inherited the coeliac gene, even if you try to shelter them, it is likely that they will be exposed to gluten at some point, which could trigger the disease later in life. There's nothing you could have done about passing on your genes.

So, how to keep your baby healthy?

It seems clear that gluten does not come through to the infant via breastmilk, and breastmilk is good for babies for all sorts of reasons. So if you can, breastfeeding is good for your baby. But it will not influence the risk of developing coeliac disease whether you breastfeed during gluten introduction or not. So feed as long as you want to, but don't do it in the hope that it will prevent coeliac disease.

When is the best time to introduce gluten?

Researchers have been investigating this for years, and have come up with mixed results.

The most recent studies (particularly from the PreventCD international research group) seem to indicate that the timing of gluten introduction does not influence the development of the disease. That is, in high risk children (children with at least one parent with coeliac disease), earlier introduction of gluten (at 4 months, vs 6 months or 12 months) is associated with earlier development of the condition, but later introduction doesn't prevent the development of coeliac disease.

How much gluten to offer?

The PreventCD researchers suggest, based on their observations, that carers should avoid giving high risk children large amounts of gluten in the first weeks after gluten introduction and during infancy. However, they have not yet established what the best introduction regime might be.

You could try introducing tiny amounts—just tastes— of gluten containing food, and gradually build it up. The advice from the Department of Health here in the UK is not to offer gluten until weaning begins at six months, and then to introduce allergens one at a time, leaving about 3 days before introducing the next new food. That way, if there is an immediate allergic response, it is clear which food is causing the problem.

Try not to worry

Use the health services available to you, whether this is a doctor, a health visitor or other medical professional. They will be able to advise you, taking into account your child's own health status and situation.

And, of course, your child has the benefit of a parent who understands about coeliac disease, and will be looking for symptoms. Just be careful not to assume that everything you see is a symptom of coeliac disease. It's very easy to assume that coeliac disease is the root cause of everything; but of course every child suffers a variety of ailments!

Practical matters

I've included documents here that I've used a number of times (sometimes editing them a bit, depending on the circumstances) with a number of different organisations, for school trips, trips with Brownies and Guides and other residentials (e.g. summer schools). I've repeated the lists of food that are (or are not) OK to eat here, to make it easier for you to use (they are given earlier in this book too).

You can download versions of these from the Free-from.com website (www.free-from.com/raising-your-coeliac-child/downloads)

Do feel free to copy them and adapt them to your own needs, replacing the words in [square brackets] where necessary.

1. Informal summary for sharing with friends
2. More formal summary for sharing with carers
3. Letter to organisation
4. List of things your child can eat
5. List of things to look out for on labels
6. Confusing or uncommon ingredients

1. Informal summary

I have coeliac disease and must eat a gluten free diet. I will be very ill if I eat gluten.

Gluten is found in wheat, barley, oats and rye, and therefore is in normal bread, pasta, cakes and biscuits. Even small amounts of gluten can make me ill.

As long as they are not cooked with wheat flour, batter, breadcrumbs or sauce, I can eat:

- rice, pulses, nuts, vegetables and fruit
- plain meat and fish
- eggs, milk and cheese.

I can eat sauces that have not been thickened with normal flour and do not contain wheat, barley, oats or rye.

Please check the ingredients for all processed food such as dressings, ketchup, stock cubes, soy sauce, burgers, sausages and spice mixes.

Please do not mix gluten free food with normal food, or prepare gluten free food using equipment used to prepare normal food without cleaning it first.

2. Formal Summary

[insert your child's name here] has been diagnosed as suffering from coeliac disease, which means **[he/she]** must eat a gluten free diet. This means no wheat, oats, barley or rye, or anything containing any derivative of these, which mostly means wheat flour. It also means most pre-prepared and processed foods and anything coated in breadcrumbs or batter, and anything containing rusk, wheat starch or modified starch. Semolina and couscous are derived from wheat.

So – **[insert your child's name here]** cannot eat standard bread, cakes, biscuits, pizza, pasta, or pastry. No chicken nuggets, fish fingers, sandwiches or pies. Gluten can be found in some brands of crisps, sweets, gravy, custard, most breakfast cereals, most sausages and burgers—the list is long. **Everything** needs to be checked. And please avoid cross-contamination with knives, spoons, pans, crumbs, and so on.

3. Letter to school, Brownies, camp, and any other event organiser

Dear [insert name of organiser],

I wanted to give you some information about catering for a child with coeliac disease. We spoke by phone last week, and you asked what **[insert your child's name here]** could eat. It is not a simple question, because everything needs to be checked, but I've come up with a list of foods that should be fine. Essentially, the less processed food on a menu, and the 'healthier' the menu, the easier it is to find something **[he/she]** can eat.

The following pages detail what **[insert your child's name here]** can/cannot eat – I hope it will be helpful to you on **[insert name of trip]**. Given that an estimated 1 in 100 people in the UK have coeliac disease, I'm sure they must have come across it before – indeed, there must be other coeliacs in school.

I'd like to reassure you that if **[he/she]** eats gluten **[he/she]** will not suffer anaphylactic shock—it isn't immediately life-threatening. However, it will damage the lining of **[his/her]** small intestine, rendering **[him/her]** less able to gain nourishment from **[his/her]** food, and **[he/she]** is likely to suffer vomiting and diarrhoea in the short term, and—if **[he/she]** ate gluten over a longer period—fatigue, inability to concentrate, ulcers, continued vomiting and diarrhoea, malnourishment and associated diseases, infertility, osteoporosis, dental problems ... the list of associated serious problems is long, so it is important that **[he/she]** remains gluten free.

If you'd like to talk through the food list, I am available by phone on **[insert tel no]** or by email on **[insert email address]**. Thank you for your help in dealing with this.

Yours truly,

[insert your own name here, and attach as much of the following information as you want]

4. List of things that are OK for coeliacs

It is a lot easier now that the food labelling has improved here in the UK, but here is a summary list of things that are likely to be OK, and things that need to be checked.

Naturally gluten free food includes:

Cereals and grains

Rice, millet, maize, quinoa, tapioca, sago, buckwheat, teff and sorghum are all gluten free

Meat, fish and eggs

These are all gluten free if unprocessed. Check any added coatings, sauces and spices, and check wafer-thin meats too (sometimes wheat flour is added to make them 'peel apart')

Dairy products

Milk, cream, butter and most cheese and yoghurt are naturally gluten free. Check any added ingredients, and check ready-grated cheese (sometimes wheat flour is added to stop the slivers of cheese sticking together). Note that blue cheese is regarded as gluten free, despite concerns some people have about the source of the mould that creates the characteristic blue veining

Flours

Rice, corn, potato, maize, gram, soya, chickpea, sorghum, tapioca and chestnut flour are all gluten free

Fruit and vegetables

Check ready-made pie fillings in case they've been thickened with flour. Check any additions such as spices, crumbles and pastry, and check any coatings, sauces and spices

Fats

Butter, margarine, oils, lard and dripping are naturally gluten free. Avoid suet unless you can find a gluten free version (it does exist, but you'll have to look for it) and do check low-fat spreads

Snacks

Nuts, raisins and seeds are naturally gluten free, but check any added coatings and check all packets of savoury snacks such as crisps (chips)

Soft drinks

Coffee, tea, juices, cocoa, fizzy drinks and most squashes are gluten free. Check that they don't contain barley or 'cloud', and don't offer drink from vending machines. Check hot chocolate, too.

Spices and seasonings

Pure salt, pepper, and herbs are naturally gluten free. Check spices and mustard powder for added flour

Vinegar

Cider, rice and wine vinegar will all be fine, but not malt vinegar, which should be avoided

Spreads and preserves

Jam, marmalade, honey and nut butters should all be naturally gluten free. Be wary of cross-contamination

Cooking ingredients

Yeast, bicarbonate of soda and cream of tartar are naturally gluten free. Check baking powder for added flour.

Available manufactured gluten free

More and more manufacturers are making gluten-free versions of 'normal' preprepared foods. Always check, but you should be able to find gluten free versions of:
- Breakfast cereals,
- Bread, crackers and crispbreads
- Cakes, pastries, cookies and biscuits
- Pizza and pasta
- Soup and sauces (check these every time, in case wheat flour has been used to thicken a soup or a sauce)
- Pies, pasties, tarts, quiche, flans
- Puddings and desserts
- Pickles, chutneys, dressings and other condiments (check these every time, because malt vinegar is

often used in pickles and soy sauce is rarely gluten free)
- Ready meals of various kinds
- Sweets (candy). Check these every time too—chocolate is usually OK to eat, but not if it covers a biscuit! All sorts of unexpected sweets contain wheat, such as Smarties, seaside rock, and licorice. Look for gluten free versions; they do exist

5. Things to look out for on labels:

Look out for the following ingredients, as these are **NOT OK** for coeliacs to eat

Atta (chapatti flour)

Barley (flakes, flour), pearl barley, pot barley, scotch barley

Bran

Breadcrumbs

Bulgar

Cereal extract

Couscous

Cracked wheat

Durum wheat

Einkorn (wheat)

Emmer (wheat)

Farina

Farro / faro

Flour

Fu—dried gluten used in some Asian dishes

Gluten

Graham flour

Kamut

Malt (extract, syrup, flavouring, vinegar, malted milk)

Modified starch (unless it states it is from a 'safe' source, e.g. rice starch or potato starch)

Matzo, matxo meal

Oat bran, oats, oatmeal, oat flour

Porridge oats, rolled oats

Rusk

Rye flour
Seitan (pure gluten)
Semolina
Spelt (this is low gluten, but not safe for coeliacs)
Triticale (a cross between wheat and rye)
Wheat bran/ wheat germ / wheat flour / wheat starch
Wholemeal flour
Wholewheat

6. Confusing or uncommon ingredients

There are some ingredients found on labels that regularly confuse people, or which are not well known. Here are a few:

Gluten free

Agar
Amaranth
Arrowroot
Buckwheat
Carageenan
Caramel
Citric acid, lactic acid, malic acid
Cornflour, cornstarch, modified corn starch
Dextrose, sucrose and fructose
Guar gum
Glucose syrup
Isomalt
Magnesium stearate
Maize, maize starch, modified maize starch
Maltodextrin
Monosodium glutamate
Polenta, sago, sorghum, tapioca, rice and quinoa
Sorbitol
Soya
Vanilla
Vegetable oils
Xanthan gum

Not Gluten Free

Barley malt
Bulgar wheat
Brewers yeast
Couscous
Licorice
Malt extract, malt syrup, malt flavouring
Malt vinegar
Pearl barley
Rusk
Semolina
Spelt
Soy sauce (unless it says gluten free)
Wheat, wheat bran, wheat rusk
Wheatgerm
Wheat starch, modified wheat starch

Thank you for reading!

Dear Reader

I hope you enjoyed Raising Your Coeliac Child, and found it useful.

I get a lot of questions via my website (free-from.com) from people just starting out on the gluten free diet—either themselves, or for their child—and I try to help where I can. This book is part of that desire to help others at what can be a very difficult stage.

Please let me know what you think: which bits helped, which bits didn't—and what I missed.

And, if you're so inclined, I'd love to read your review of Raising Your Coeliac Child on Amazon. Please be honest; I'd like to know what could be improved, as well as what you liked. And your review might make all the difference to whether someone else who needs this information finds the book online.

Thank you so much for reading!

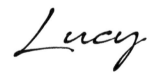

Lucy lives in rural England with her husband and their three children. The eldest was diagnosed with coeliac disease as a one-year-old, so the family have all been dealing with the gluten free diet for over twenty years— and have survived everything from school dinners and childhood birthday parties to Guide camps, Duke of Edinburgh expeditions and travelling abroad.

Twenty years ago, there wasn't much support for parents of coeliac children, so Lucy set up and ran a support group for local coeliac children as part of the local Coeliac UK group.

In 2006 she set up a website at free-from.com to continue to share what she's learned about living gluten free. Her blog was identified in 2011 as one of the UK's top 5 allergy blogs.

More recently, she's served for several years on the judging panel for the Free From Food Awards and for the Free From Eating Out Awards.

Index